DIAGNOSTIC PULMONARY CYTOLOGY

Geno Saccomanno, PhD, MD
Pathologist
St. Mary's Hospital and Medical Center
Veterans Administration Hospital
Grand Junction, Colorado

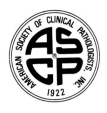

Educational Products Division
American Society of Clinical Pathologists
Chicago

Library of Congress Cataloging in Publication Data
Saccomanno, Geno, 1915–
    Diagnostic pulmonary cytology.
    Bibliography:
    Includes index.
    1. Lungs—Cancer—Diagnosis—Atlases. 2. Diagnosis, Cytologic—Atlases.
3. Exfoliative cytology—Atlases. 4. Sputum—Examination—Atlases. I. Title.
[DNLM: 1. Cytodiagnosis—Atlases. 2. Lung neoplasms—Diagnosis—Atlases.
3. Lung—Cytology—Atlases. WF17 S119d]
RC280.L8S23   616.9′94′24   78-8285
ISBN 0-89189-050-5

DIAGNOSTIC PULMONARY CYTOLOGY

To my wife, Virginia, for her patience, love, and understanding.

TABLE OF CONTENTS

PREFACE

The primary objective of this text is to aid the cytotechnology student, the cytotechnologist, and the cytopathologist in the diagnosis of cancer of the lung. The cellular elements seen on slides prepared from sputum samples and pleural aspirates are shown by color photography. In addition to the cytological photographs, histological sections of most of the tumors are presented. The purpose of this presentation is to establish clearly the similarities and differences between the results of these two methods of studying pulmonary tumors. Often, the histology reveals the most common cell forming the tumor but this may or may not be the same as the cell most commonly identified on the smear.

All cells found in sputum — normal, inflammatory, premalignant, and malignant — have been indexed and catalogued so that the student can readily compare cells discussed in the text with those seen under the microscope. The details of collection, preparation, and staining methods are presented as lucidly as possible, and the importance of each of these phases is stressed.

The first eight plates show cells that represent the response of the lung both to acute and chronic inflammation, with discussion of the function of these cells and the frequency with which they are seen. Specific cell patterns in some diseases are demonstrated to assist in the identification of all cells present on the smear prepared from sputum.

Plates 9–15 are devoted to the histology and cytology of squamous cell metaplasia. Frequently, these cells are misdiagnosed as neoplasia and are poorly understood with regard to cause and significance; therefore, they are presented and classified on the basis of varying degrees of atypia.

Plates 16–44 demonstrate the histology and cytology of the most common tumors of the lung. Care has been taken to match the color of Papanicolaou or other good stains so that the same cellular features can be seen under the microscope. The student can readily find all neoplastic cells on the plates for comparison. An attempt has been made on most plates to present a wide range of cell patterns. These are discussed in detail.

Plates 45 and 46 show two interesting cases of mesothelioma with discussion of their behavior. Plates 47–65 demonstrate metastatic sputum cells and histological sections of the tumor exfoliating these cells. As a consequence of the advent of chemotherapy, advanced carcinogenesis is receiving more and more attention. In some cases, sputum cytology serves as an adequate monitor of chemotherapeutic response. This method of monitoring may prove even more effective as new anticarcinogenic drugs are found.

This work represents an effort to facilitate visual comparison of cells shown in the plates with those seen through the microscope on well-prepared, well-stained sputum slides. The purpose of this book, then, is to further early diagnosis, resulting in better patient care and increased patient survival.

ACKNOWLEDGMENTS

This text is the product of many dedicated persons interested in the constant improvement of care of the cancer patient. To those who contributed to this task, I am very grateful. Mr Jerry Scott, CT (ASCP), photographer, contributed to the selection of cases from a cytological viewpoint, painstakingly photographed most of them and arranged the plates. His meticulous attention to detail speaks for itself. Mrs Lola Brennan, BS, CT (ASCP), Chief Cytotechnologist, St Mary's Hospital and Medical Center, assisted in selecting cases, researching materials, and reading the manuscript. Obviously, all of the students and cytotechnologists in St Mary's Department of Cytopathology contributed to this èffort. The Department of Energy (Contract No. EY-76-C-02-1826) and the US Public Health Service and their representatives, particularly Joseph Goldstein, MD, Walter Weyzen, MD (Present Medical Director, Department of Energy, Washington, DC), and Victor Archer, MD deserve thanks for help in gaining financial support and for their constant encouragement. I acknowledge Oscar Auerbach, MD for his help and contribution of specimens from the Uranium Miner Lung Study. The staff members of St Mary's Department of Pathology, Drs R.P. Saunders, M.G. Klein, and J. Steinbrecher, are to be thanked for their encouragement and patience. The administrators, the physicians, and the patients both at St Mary's Hospital and at the Veterans Administration Hospital in Grand Junction, Colorado deserve thanks for their contributions. The editorial staff at the American Society of Clinical Pathologists was helpful and diligent in the preparation of the manuscript for final printing. And, finally, but not least, Mrs Willie L. Turner, secretary, deserves special thanks for her contribution in proofreading and typing.

DIAGNOSTIC PULMONARY CYTOLOGY

INTRODUCTION

PULMONARY CYTOLOGY

Cancer of the lung is the most common malignant neoplasm among the American male population[1] and is a rapidly increasing malignant lesion in the female population as well. Historically, cancer of the lung was an almost unheard of disease in the 18th century and a rarity in the 19th century.[2, 3] The rarity of these tumors and the absence of X-rays and tissue sections, which were not available until the early part of the 19th century, made the differentiation between inflammatory diseases and neoplasia of the lung very difficult if not impossible. Virchow[4] was one of the first scientists to utilize cellular identification of tumors by microscopy in the diagnosis of lung lesions.

The first microscopic description of cancer of the lung was made by Quain in 1857.[5] The metastases from these lesions were first reported by Greene[6] in 1843. Bronchoscopy with direct visualization of the tracheobronchial tree, made possible for the first time by Killian,[7] completed the triad of histology, X-ray, and visual observation of the main bronchi, which aided in differentiating neoplasia from inflammatory diseases. At that time, tuberculosis was probably the most common chronic lung disease that had to be differentiated from lung neoplasia. Today, of course, the reverse is the case. Tumor is common, and tuberculosis is a rare lesion of the lung, at least in this country. With increased cigarette smoking and exposure to other respiratory carcinogens, a neoplasm of the lung rare in the previous century has become the most common in man today.

As the incidence of cancer of the lung increased, radiological diagnosis improved. Anesthesia and surgical treatment developed rapidly; nonetheless, the five-year survival period stabilized at only 5%, much less than expected. Even though our knowledge about these tumors increased, the response remained poor. It then became apparent that when lesions were large enough to be seen radiologically they were, in reality, in an advanced state of development and, all too frequently, had already spread to regional nodes and other areas. Means of identifying the incipient stages of tumor development became possible with the advent of sputum cytology.[8]

The art of sputum cytological diagnosis was not available during the first half of the 20th century. Papanicolaou, the father of modern cytology, presented his first case of the cytological diagnosis of lung cancer in 1945.[9] Although occasional cytological diagnoses had been reported previously, Papanicolaou was the first to use cytology for identification of these lesions, which initiated the technique as a worthwhile procedure.

With better techniques of sputum collection, preservation, and preparation, the diagnosis of lung cancer improved and sputum cytology became common in the modern hospital laboratory. Moreover, pulmonary cytology has become an accepted method of screening in the identification of the effects of single and multiple carcinogens in high-risk populations. Metastatic malignancies to the lung are also readily identified by sputum cytology, which will prove to be valuable in monitoring advanced disease, particularly in assessing the effectiveness of chemotherapy.

1

Fiberoptic bronchoscopy has contributed materially to the localization of lung tumors. This method enables the diagnosis of very small, as well as large, lesions. With continued research, it should allow localization of early in situ cancer of the lung and improve the five-year survival period.[10]

All of these methods of diagnosis and treatment of lung cancer are, at present, poorly integrated and probably not yielding much improvement in the five-year survival period. However, all of these techniques are being improved rapidly and will contribute tremendously in the near future. Many novel ideas in immunology, fluorescence,[11] fiberoptics, and cytotechnology show much promise in this field.

Keratinizing epidermoid cancer of the lung, the most common lung carcinoma, is readily diagnosed in sputum smears because of bizarre cytological patterns and an abundance of tumor cells. Many of the other cancers of the lung, however, are difficult to diagnose because of subtle cellular patterns, fewer cells, and rarity as lung lesions.

It is the object of this text to present cases and discussions which, it is hoped, will provide a ready reference to the student in cytotechnology training, the cytotechnologist, and cytopathologist. The squamous and adenocarcinomas of the lung vary markedly, histologically and cytologically; therefore, where justified, several tumors of each type are presented to familiarize the student with these variants. Using histological and cytological photographs, this work presents premalignant and malignant tumor cells found in the sputum and originating in primary and metastatic tumors of the lung.

REFERENCES

1. Silverberg E: Cancer statistics, 1977. CA 27:26–41, 1977
2. Morgagni JB: De sedibus et causi morborum. Lavanii Typogr. Acad., 1761, Lib. II, ep. 22 (quoted by Pepper[3])
3. Pepper W: Cases of cancer of the lungs and mediastinum. Trans Stud Coll Physicians Phila 1:96–110, 1850
4. Virchow R: Cellular Pathology. London: J. Churchill, 1860, p 479
5. Quain F: Encephaloid tumor involving the heart and lungs. Br Med J 44:902, 1857
6. Greene S: Encephaloid tumours in the brain and lungs. Dublin J Med Sci 24:282–283, 1843
7. Killian G: Uber Directe Bronchoskopie. Munch Med Wochenschr 45:844–874, 1898
8. Saccomanno G, et al: Cancer of the lung; the cytology of sputum prior to the development of carcinoma. Acta Cytol 9:413–423, 1965
9. Papanicolaou GN: Diagnostic value of exfoliated cells from cancerous tissues. JAMA 131:372–378, 1946
10. Woolner LB, et al: In-situ and early invasive bronchogenic carcinoma: report of 28 cases with post-operative survival data. J Thorac Cardiovasc Surg 60:275, 1970
11. Profio AE, Doiron DR: A feasibility study of the use of fluorescence bronchoscopy for localization of small lung tumors. Phys Med Biol 22:949–957, 1977

MATERIALS AND METHODS

The field of pulmonary cytology embraces many phases of technology which must be integrated to yield ideal results. The quality and quantity of the specimen are dependent on collection, preservation, preparation, staining, and screening, which are some of the phases of sputum cytology that must be handled carefully, or the end product will be inadequate for a correct diagnosis. Each step is a link in a chain, which is only as strong as its weakest link. Obviously, if the sample collected is inadequate, not primarily of lung origin, the correct diagnosis will not be possible even after efficient processing. If the fixative is inadequate, although the sample may be directly from the tumor, and the processing, staining, and reading are done very efficiently, the cells will be degenerated, making an accurate diagnosis impossible. Every step in the process must be perfect if a definitive diagnosis is to be made. A detailed description[1] of the collection, preparation, staining, and reading of material is given in the next section.

In the assessment of sputum slide material, the student is encouraged to identify all cells seen in the smear. Recognition of the presence or absence of tumor cells is the primary objective of the proper reading of a sputum smear; however, recognition of all cells present will elicit other worthwhile information. The amount of inflammation present allows assessment of the presence and degree of chronic obstructive pulmonary disease.[2] The presence of eosinophils admixed in the exudate may reveal an allergic reaction or Löffler's syndrome(see Plate 8). The identification of the various degrees of squamous metaplasia gives some assessment of premalignant cellular changes in the bronchial tree and indirectly suggests the degree of carcinogenic exposure or sensitivity of the patient to a particular carcinogen.

Identification of all cellular elements is encouraged throughout this text and played an important role in the selection of material for photography. The presence of macrophages and tall columnar cells indicates that the specimen is of lung origin; therefore one must be constantly aware of these cellular elements to ensure that the specimen is indeed of lung origin and adequate. Unsatisfactory specimens always leave a void—the patient may have a malignancy, but the diagnosis cannot be made. It is important to evaluate a specimen properly, and if it is inadequate in some way, that should be acknowledged. It is misleading to call a specimen satisfactory when it is not, because this gives the physician a false sense of security. Evaluation of the various qualities of each specimen are discussed.

The most common lesions of the lungs, larynx, and pleura are presented in this text and shown histologically and cytologically. Examination of the tissue sections frequently reveals characteristics which may shed light on the cytology. Variations of cell size and arrangement, preservation, and necrosis of cells are seen most vividly in tissues and account for many of the variations noted cytologically. For example, when one examines a section of malignant tumor, one notes that the cell size varies markedly, but it is still obvious that all of the cells in the tumor are components of it. While examining a smear on which cells are scattered, one tends to be impressed with the larger cells, frequently discounting smaller ones. The same consideration applies to the nuclear/

3

cytoplasmic (N/C) ratio. Cells with increased N/C ratio attract attention readily, while those with a normal N/C ratio, even though having all the other features of malignancy, are not nearly as impressive and may be overlooked.

Of course, the cytology of a lesion is most important because it is the only element available for establishing the diagnosis. Most of the frames in this text are of cytology, and an attempt is made to show as wide a variety of cells as possible. Particular attention, wherever possible, is paid to cell size. The cells were not accurately measured but were estimated by comparison to polymorphonuclear leukocytes, which measure about 8–9 μ in diameter. Cell size is a very important tool, since some cells are similar in all observable characteristics such as cytoplasm, staining, and nuclear features, except size. Note some of the cells in the undifferentiated epidermoid tumors in Plates 24, 25, and 27 and compare these with the tumor cells seen in some of the oat cell carcinomas in Plates 41 and 42. Size of cells is a very important distinguishing feature in the identification of these tumors.

The cytological photographs are intended to simulate, as closely as possible, the cells seen microscopically in sputum under a 15× ocular in both low and high power. The commentary on the opposite page gives age and smoking history when this is important. Some comments about X-rays are also included when pertinent to the discussion as well as remarks about salient features of the histology. In the discussion of the cells, an attempt is made to orient the reader to size and staining features, with emphasis on the features that contribute to the diagnosis of a benign cell pattern or malignant tumor. Particular attention is paid to the features of the nucleus, because frequently it is well preserved while the cytoplasm is degenerate.

Most of the specimens selected for presentation in this text were collected from inpatients and outpatients at St Mary's and Veterans Administration Hospitals. The histological material is from lung biopsies, resected lesions of the lung, or from autopsies. The remaining specimens were collected in the course of the uranium miner lung study on the Colorado Plateau. This study has been in progress for 20 years and involves the collection of sputum samples and tissue from miners who developed cancer of the lung. Many of these patients had provided sputum samples for several years prior to the development of cancer. These studies have proven worthwhile, particularly in developing insight on how tumors develop in the premalignant as well as malignant stages. It is of interest to mention here that cancer of the lung in uranium miners is no different in its development from tumors that develop in cigarette smokers, except that the addition of the second carcinogen (radiation) results in a slight increase in the incidence of small cell tumors of the lung.[3, 4, 5]

Whenever possible, the tissue sections are from the same tumor that released the cells collected in the sputum. When this was not possible, matching of tumor and cell types was made to show similar patterns. All of the tissue sections were stained with Mayer's hematoxylin and eosin (H&E). All sputum samples were prepared with the Saccomanno technique[6] and stained with Papanicolaou stain. All photographs were taken with a Zeiss photomicroscope II on Kodacolor-X and Kodacolor II film and printed on Kodak paper. The photos were taken with Planapo 40 oil immersion objective, resulting in a magnification of ×600. A 6.3 × Neofluar objective was used for the low-power ×100 magnification and a Planapo objective was used for the medium magnification of ×400. As mentioned elsewhere, all cells can readily be measured by comparison with the size of a polymorphonuclear leukocyte or lymphocyte, which average between $8-10\ \mu$.

REFERENCES

1. Saccomanno G: Sputum cytology: collection, fixation, and concentration of sputum, bronchial aspirates, and bronchial brushings. ASCP Technical Improvement Service, No. 27, 1976
2. Mittman C, Stevens D, Teplitz R: Cellular elements in sputum as an index of obstructive lung disease. (Unpublished)
3. Auerbach O, et al: Changes in the bronchial epithelium in relation to smoking and cancer of the lung. N Engl J Med 256:97−104, 1957
4. Saccomanno G, et al: Cancer of the lung; the cytology of sputum prior to the development of carcinoma. Acta Cytol 9:413−423, 1965
5. Saccomanno G, et al: Development of carcinoma of the lung as reflected in exfoliated cells. Cancer 33:256−270, 1974
6. Saccomanno G, et al: Concentration of carcinoma or atypical cells in sputum. Acta Cytol 7:305−310, 1963

SPUTUM CYTOLOGY: COLLECTION, FIXATION, AND CONCENTRATION OF SPUTUM, BRONCHIAL ASPIRATES, AND BRONCHIAL BRUSHINGS

CLINICAL RATIONALE

Normally, the epithelium of the tracheobronchial tree has a total cellular turnover of 30 days.[1] This turnover results in an abundance of epithelial cellular discharge in the lumen of the bronchial tree. Many of these cells degenerate, fragment, and are not found in the expectorated sputum. Many, however, are found in the sputum in various stages of preservation. Some appear normal, others show fragmentation and swelling, and many may simulate tumor cells. Inflammatory cells are usually abundant, particularly in bronchitis, and may also be well preserved and/or degenerated. Effects of inflammation and respiratory carcinogens also cause cellular changes in the respiratory epithelium.

The lining cells of the tracheobronchial tree respond in a variety of ways to inflammation and exposure to respiratory carcinogens throughout long periods. This epithelium undergoes hyperplasia in the initial periods of insult, but if this is prolonged, be it inflammation or carcinogen, areas of squamous cell metaplasia develop. Initially, these areas of squamous cell metaplasia are usually small. They are most frequently noted on the bronchial spurs, extending for very short distances and are either abruptly or gradually joined by normal, tall columnar cells. With continued exposure, these areas of metaplasia increase in size and gradually become more and more cytologically atypical. In a few cases,[2] they may eventually become malignant.

During this process of tumorigenesis, the epithelium, normal and abnormal, continues to shed cells into the sputum and is subject to cytological examination. A sputum sample that is of lung origin will therefore show a variety of cells representative of what is actually being shed by the lung lining at that time. If metaplasia is present, metaplastic cells are found in the sputum. If tumor is present, tumor cells will be found in the sputum, so that a sputum sample is a good index of what is being shed from the whole bronchial tree. Tumors, however, develop in isolated areas, and the problem then becomes one of localization of the lesion. Roentgenograms of the chest are helpful if the lesion is large enough to be seen; however, this is a late finding. Localization of lesions smaller than those visible on X-ray film is difficult, necessitating direct visualization with rigid or fiberoptic bronchoscopy. Confirmation with either tissue biopsy or smear specimens from the suspicious area can then be made. Therefore, a variety of specimens must be examined, depending on such factors as the presence or absence of neoplasia and the size of the lesion. The specimens to be examined consist of the following: (1) sputum, to determine the degree of disease present; (2) bronchial washings, used in an attempt to localize the lesion to a specific lung or lobe; (3) bronchial brushings, to assess abnormal-appearing areas; and (4) biopsy tissue, taken from areas suspected of having tumor. These various specimens and their manner of preparation will be described separately.

SPUTUM COLLECTION, PRESERVATION, AND PREPARATION OF SLIDES FOR CYTOLOGICAL STUDY

The object is to collect a satisfactory amount of sputum of pulmonary origin. The patient should not only be informed that it is essential that an adequate amount of sputum is necessary but should also be given some information on the physiology and anatomy of the respiratory system, with detailed instructions that the sputum needed must come from "deep in the lungs." One must explain that such materials as nasal aspirates and tongue scrapings, not being of pulmonary origin, are not what is desired. Sometimes this is a difficult point to put across, particularly if the patient is frightened or anxious about the diagnosis. The patient must be at ease with the person explaining the procedure, whether that is collection of a sputum sample the following morning or presently the use of an aerosol. It has been our experience that patients are frequently so worried that they hear little of the instructions and must be put at ease. Following the instructions, it is sometimes worthwhile to ask patients direct questions to confirm that they know what you are talking about. Once the patient knows what is desired, the specimen can be collected in two ways: at home on first arising from bed or by use of an aerosol. The collection of sputum at home will be discussed first.

Usually, patients with diagnostic lung problems are cigarette smokers and, after the discussion on the type of sputum sample desired, know exactly what is needed. They will readily admit that on arising from bed they cough up material from deep in the lungs. A rare person, although a cigarette smoker, will not be able to produce sufficient cough material for study, but 90% of all patients will yield a satisfactory specimen spontaneously on arising from a night's sleep. The remaining 10% of the patients who do not cough must be administered an aerosol.

EARLY MORNING SPECIMENS FOR PULMONARY CYTOLOGICAL EXAMINATION

The patient is given three wide-mouthed specimen bottles, each containing 50 ml of fixative, consisting of 48 ml of 50% ethyl alcohol diluted from 95% ethyl alcohol, to which has been added 1 ml of 50% polyethylene glycol (Carbowax 1540) (Union Carbide Corporation, New York, NY) and 1 ml of ethyl alcohol containing 3 mg of Rifampin (Dow Chemical Company, Midland, MI). It should be explained that this is not a potable alcohol and must be used for fixation only. Staining material, such as eosin or methylene blue, may be added to prevent drinking of the fixative. The patients are instructed to use one container each morning, not adding more than 15–20 ml or the equivalent of four or five tablespoons of sputum. They are instructed to rinse their mouths with water on arising. One of the bottles should be available, and, on coughing, the patient should spit into the bottle, firmly tighten the lid, and shake vigorously for a few seconds. The procedure is repeated until the estimated amount of four to five tablespoons of sputum is added to the bottle. This is done for three consecutive mornings. These three specimens are returned to the laboratory for processing, where they are pooled into one.

The noncoughing patients are administered an aerosol (Fig. 1 on p 11), which may be accomplished in the following manner. Various aerosol instruments can be used. When available, we prefer the one by DeVilbiss (Toledo, OH); however, the Monaghan Ultrasonic Nebulizer (Pueblo, CO) can be used. The object of aerosolization is to introduce a significant amount of water into the lungs. Irritants or mucolytic agents can be added, but our experience with these has not yielded any improvement over tap water. It is most important again to explain to the patient the procedure and the expected result. After 20 to 30 minutes of aerosol inspiration, the patient should take at least four deep breaths, and on the fifth, forcefully attempt to cough. This procedure should be repeated with reasonable rest periods between attempts. Sometimes, if the patient cannot produce an adequate sample using an aerosol, he will have a productive cough within the next 24 hours. Therefore, the patient should be given a bottle containing fixative and instructions for collecting a sputum sample during this period of time. The sputum specimen should always be collected after the patient washes his or her mouth with water. The specimen is expectorated into a large-mouth bottle, about half full of 50% ethyl alcohol (95% ethyl alcohol diluted to 50%; do not use absolute), containing 1 ml of 50% polyethylene glycol (Carbowax 1540) and 1 ml of 50% ethyl alcohol containing 3 mg of Rifampin.

PROCESSING OF FIXED SPUTUM SAMPLES COLLECTED SPONTANEOUSLY OR WITH AN AEROSOL

It should be mentioned that the fixative of 50% ethyl alcohol plus Carbowax has been found to adequately sterilize the specimens in our laboratory; however, it is advised that we are adding 1 ml of 50% ethyl alcohol containing 3 mg of Rifampin to the fixative in each bottle prior to collection. On arrival of the specimen at the laboratory, another equal amount of Rifampin is added. The specimen is processed after 24 hours. If a negative pressure hood is available, the blending should be done in the hood. These are added precautions that should be taken, particularly if the specimens are from populations showing a high incidence of mycobacteria. In areas of high incidence of pathogenic fungi, antifungal amphotericin B should probably be added to the fixative before processing.

PROCEDURE

The specimen bottle lid is removed, and visual inspection of the sample is made to note its color and coarseness, or whether it is composed of large mucous blobs. This is important in assessing the blending time. If the material is pale and cloudy, the blending can be kept to a minimum; if large mucous blobs or thick masses of brown material are noted, then blending must be longer. Blending does not fragment cells but does create currents that, at 22,000 rpm, allow most of the fine mucous fibers to liquify and partly dissolve the larger fibers, though some are cut and will be seen as segments of mucous fibers on the smear. The bottle containing the sputum is emptied into the blending vessel (Fig. 2 on p 11), on which a lid is placed and which is then inserted into the blender. Blending should be complete and adequate in three to four seconds for most specimens. When the cap is removed, visual examination of the specimen will reveal a homogeneous, cloudy liquid. If coarse particles are noted, the specimen should be blended for another two or three seconds. The blended sputum is then poured into 50-ml plastic or glass test tubes (10 cm in length and 22–26 mm in diameter) for centrifuging (Fig. 3 on p 11).

Note that between specimens the blender chamber is washed with hot running water with several rinses until a foam stops forming (Fig. 4 on p 11). Because the chamber has a smooth surface, no carryover cells have been found experimentally. The specimens are then centrifuged (Fig. 5 on p 11) at 1,500 rpm for 15 minutes, and the supernatant material is decanted (Fig. 6 on p 11). This is a critical point because if the centrifugate is abundant, less fluid should be decanted than if a small amount of material is noted. Enough fluid should remain so that on vibrating the tube (Fig. 7 on p 11) sufficient liquid is present to allow the centrifugate to be suspended in the fluid. Too much fluid will result in a very thin smear, and too little will result in a thick slide preparation. The vibrating of the tube is done for only a few seconds. If a vibrator is not available, the tubes can be agitated by snapping the side of the tube with a flip of one's finger.

Once the specimen is vibrated, either an aspirator pipette may be used or the large tube can be everted, allowing about two drops to fall on a properly labeled slide (Fig. 8 on p 11). Another slide is placed over the specimen, and the two slides with the two drops of sputum matrix are then worked in a sliding manner until the material appears to be distributed uniformly into a thin film over the slides. The slides are then pulled apart along the long axis and are allowed to dry for at least an hour before staining. These slides can also be kept in this stage for not more than 2 to 3 days before staining. Excessive drying, however, can cause cell shrinkage. It is thought that the Carbowax forms a cellular coating, which prevents cellular shrinkage. The slides are then stained with Papanicolaou's stain, after fixation for 10 minutes in 95% alcohol, followed by a five-minute wash in running tap water (Fig. 9 on p 11). The staining procedure follows. Three control slides are checked by the laboratory supervisor daily for quality of stains.

STAINING PROCEDURE FOR SPUTUM SMEARS

1. Post-fix sputum specimen in 95% ethyl alcohol (ROH) for 10 minutes.
2. Rinse in running tap water for five minutes.
3. Stain with hematoxylin for one minute.
4. Rinse under running tap water until the water is clear.
5. Immerse in 95% ROH two times for one minute each.
6. Stain with OG-6 (Ortho Pharmaceutical Corp., Raritan, NJ) for two and one-half minutes.
7. Agitate in 95% ROH three times for one minute each time.

8. Stain with EA-36 or EA-50 (Ortho Pharmaceutical Corp.) for one and one-half minutes.
9. Agitate in 95% ROH three times for one minute each time.
10. Rinse in absolute alcohol two times for one minute each time.
11. Clear in xylene, three changes (five minutes minimum), until specimen is ready for cover glass.

BRONCHIAL ASPIRATES AND BRONCHIAL BRUSHINGS

The personnel responsible for preparing specimens originating from bronchial washings or brushings are from the cytology department at our hospital. Our experience has taught us that the bronchoscopist and other people in the surgery suite are busy with the performance of their tasks and too frequently are unable to prepare and properly fix samples. In any case, the cytotechnologists perform the cytologic screening and will, after all, do a better job than the surgeon who appreciates their help and, being released from slide preparation responsibilities, can better perform his or her duties.

The bronchial aspirates are collected in 50% ethyl alcohol and Carbowax, and are subsequently taken to the cytology laboratory to be prepared like the fixed sputum samples. Four slides are prepared on each aspirated sample.

BRONCHIAL BRUSHINGS

We have found that the disposable brushes yield an excellent sample if all of the cells on the brush are recovered. This is done in the following manner: As the bronchoscopist withdraws the brush from the bronchoscope, it is immediately handed to the cytotechnologist, who cuts the wire with scissors, leaving only about 4 inches of wire attached. The surgeon must be certain to advise the cytotechnologist exactly from which bronchus the brush has been withdrawn. The cytotechnologist marks the slides, identifying the sample, and makes the smear on the slide, which is immediately immersed in 95% ethyl alcohol in a Coplin jar. The cytotechnologist then inserts the brush in the fixative of 50% ethyl alcohol and Carbowax described previously. The brush is then agitated vigorously in the fixative. This solution, containing cells from the brush (brush wash), is centrifuged without blending. Smears are made, allowed to dry, and stained with Papanicolaou's procedure as described before.

REFERENCES

1. Naib ZM: Exfoliative Cytopathology, ed 2. Boston: Little, Brown and Co., 1976
2. Saccomanno G, et al: Development of carcinoma of the lung as reflected in exfoliated cells. Cancer 33:256–270, 1974
3. Saccomanno G, et al: Concentration of carcinoma or atypical cells in sputum. Acta Cytol 7:305–310, 1963

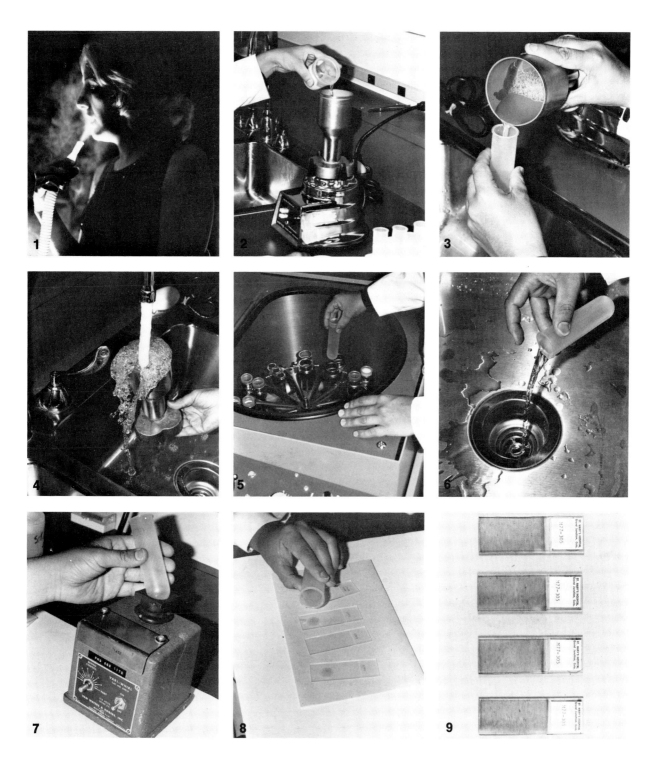

Figures 1—9. Sputum collection, preservation, and preparation of slides for cytological study.

Plate 1

SPUTUM SMEARS

The slides prepared for cytological screening of sputum material must be prepared to yield a uniform distribution of cells. The cells must be of sufficient concentration to cover nearly all areas and still reveal a minimal amount of overlap. Needless to say, the material must be blended enough to interrupt the mucous fibers but not so excessively as to cause some cellular destruction. Most of the cells in sputum samples from patients without upper respiratory infection or chronic bronchitis are squamous. These are flat and readily recognized. Histiocytes and other cells usually gravitate to the intermingling areas and are easily identified. Figure 1 is a low power view of a smear revealing an adequate distribution of cell components. Figures 2–6 are high power views and reveal proper staining and cell distribution.

This method of sputum preparation results in adequate distribution and ideal staining with Papanicolaou stain,[1] and it concentrates cell elements about 20:1.[2]

REFERENCES

1. Papanicolaou GN: Atlas of Exfoliative Cytology. Cambridge, MA: Harvard University Press, 1954
2. Ellis D, Kernosky JJ: Efficiency of concentrating malignant cells in sputum. Acta Cytologica 7:372–373, 1963

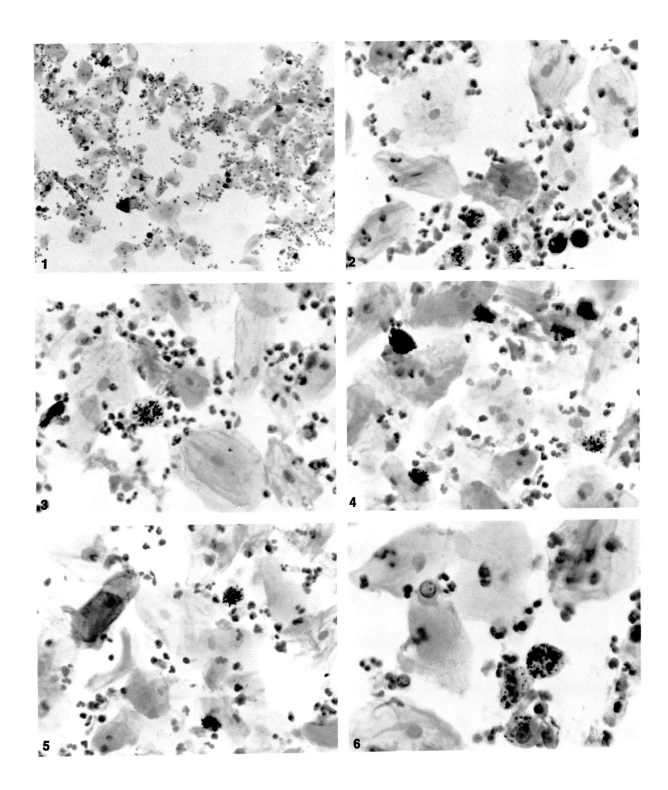

Plate 2

HISTIOCYTES (MACROPHAGES, DUST CELLS)

For diagnostic purposes, identification of histiocytes in their various stages of development is important, because they are sometimes confused with tumor cells. Histiocytes can engulf endogenous and exogenous products, but this does not alter the cells materially, except that the more material they engulf the larger they become. The engulfed material then aids to identify the cells as histiocytes. All histiocytes originate from fixed histiocytes or from the blood stream, are seen in abundance in the alveolar spaces and the bronchial tree, and are easily found in sputum samples.

Young histiocytes, as well as some that show early macrophage activity, will be discussed here. These cells are present in all exudate material of the respiratory tract but, as mentioned above, are more abundantly seen in the alveolar spaces. Since these areas are lined by flattened alveolar cells that do not have cilia to move metabolic debris, histiocytes apparently perform the task. How these cells migrate out of the alveolar areas and the tracheobronchial tree is still not completely understood, but they are forever present in this area and certainly must play an important role. The young histiocytes contain little cytoplasm and show no engulfed material in it (Figs. 1–7). The nuclei of these cells are usually round but may be elongated (Figs. 1–7) or kidney shaped (Fig. 6). The nuclear material is finely granular with one, two, or three chromocenters (Figs. 3,4). Frequently, if the nucleus is flat, a slightly angled depression or cleft is noted along the nuclear border. This sometimes molds the nucleus into a kidney shape. On occasion, a large aggregate of these cells is noted, forming a huge pseudogiant cell (Fig. 2). These differ from true giant cells in that there is no giant cell membrane. Note that these cells seem to be suspended or aggregated by a fine basophilic mucous matrix, which also houses some polymorphonuclear leukocytes. Cells in Figure 8 show engulfed lipid or some other substance that forms a vacuole. The nuclei of the adjacent cells are very similar although there is marked variance of cell size. Other vacuolated cells are seen in Figures 9 and 11. The cells in Figure 10 have phagocytized a greenish substance, while those in Figure 12 are more mature and show more cytoplasm with only granulations in the cytoplasm of some of them.

14

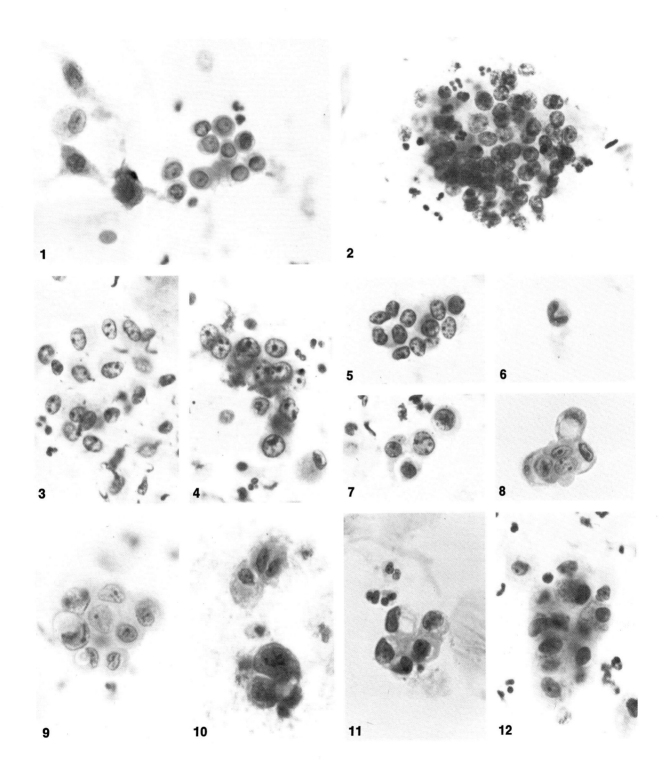

Plate 3

HISTIOCYTES (MACROPHAGES, DUST CELLS)

These histiocytes are readily recognized as a group of cells that contain abundant engulfed material in their cytoplasm. The three cells in the center of the frame in Figure 1 contain a yellow-green material. Those in Figure 3 contain black carbonaceous substance. The cells in Figure 6 contain yellow-orange hemosiderin of lysed red cell origin.[1,2] The histiocytes in Figures 7–10 contain lipid-like substance. This could be studied with fat stains.[3] All of these cells are enlarged, measuring from 20 to 60 μ in diameter. The nuclei are obscured by the engulfed material and some have been pushed to the margins of the cells.

REFERENCES

1. Gomori G: Micro-technical demonstration of iron: a criticism of its methods. Am J Pathol 12:655–663, 1936
2. Bridges CH, Luna LG: Kerr's improved Warthin-Starry technic; study of the permissible variations. Lab Invest 6:357–367, 1957
3. Luna, LG: Oil red "O" in propylene glycol method for fats, in Manual of Histologic Staining Methods, ed. 3. Washington, DC: AFIP, 1968, pp. 140–142

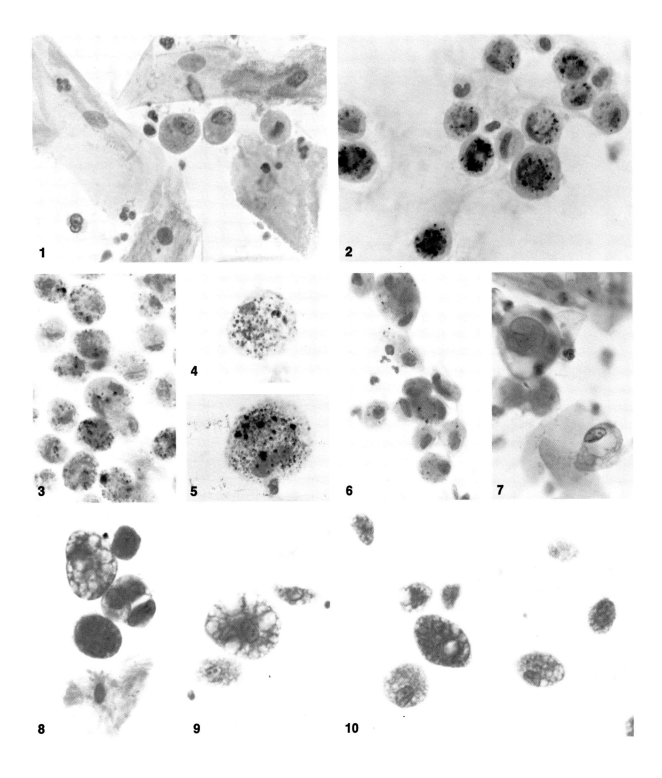

Plate 4

MORPHOLOGY OF ABNORMAL SPUTUM

This plate is divided into three sections. The upper section reveals the effects of blending the fixed sputum sample. Sputum is composed of two elements. The first element discussed is mucus, and the second consists of cells found in sputum. The mucous fibers vary in size from very fine fibers to thick long strands. A thick section of a mucous fiber is seen in Figure 3. Figures 1 and 2 show thinner fibers. The object of blending is to create rapid currents in the specimen that literally dissolve or resuspend the small fine mucous fibers in solution. The larger fibers are reduced considerably in size, and some of the large thick fibers are cut into sections, as seen in Figure 3. Other smaller fibers are seen distributed throughout Figures 1 and 2. The second element, of course, consists of the cells, both fixed and free, that are found in sputum. Normally, only histiocytes, leukocytes (free cells), and squamous metaplastic cells (fixed) form most of these elements, but in disease, other cells are added, such as neoplastic cells, which are the essence of this text.

The middle section of this plate shows an abundance of acute inflammatory cells. In severe chronic obstructive pulmonary disease, there is a marked increase in exudate and this consists predominantly of polymorphonuclear inflammatory cells (pus cells). Often, abundant bacteria are admixed with these cells, as free bacteria or as clusters. Obviously, smears in which inflammatory cells predominate are markedly diluted by these elements and result in little or no concentration, with less chance of revealing tumor cells. Occasionally, a tumor cell is found in a specimen (Fig. 7), but often these cells are markedly degenerated. This always necessitates another sputum sample, which is rarely better than the one that housed the degenerated tumor cell. Nonetheless, these specimens have to be read or screened in their entirety lest tumor cells be missed. Obviously, a diagnosis of infectious, acute suppurative bronchitis is made. This condition is known clinically as chronic obstructive pulmonary disease and is usually one of the complications of clinical diseases of chronic cigarette smoking with resultant emphysema, pulmonary fibrosis, etc. Treating these patients with high doses of antibiotics decreases the inflammatory disease, and the quality of the sputum sample following therapy in these cases improves. Approximately 10% of sputum samples from high-risk patients will reveal an abundance of inflammatory cells.

The third group of frames show Curschmann's spirals. These are fibers of proteinaceous material from distant bronchioles that project into the respiratory alveoli. These mucous bodies are of many configurations, have hairy surfaces, vary in width and length, and often are quite tortuous, as demonstrated in Figures 8–11. Some writers[1] have demonstrated tumor cells in these proteinaceous fibers. We have not been able to find that these structures yield cells that are not usually abundant in the smear anyway.

REFERENCE

1. Fullmer CD, et al: Sputum of chronic cigarette smokers. Microscopic observations and incidence of bronchial and bronchiolar spirals, fibrils, and casts. Rocky M Med J 66: 42–46, 1969

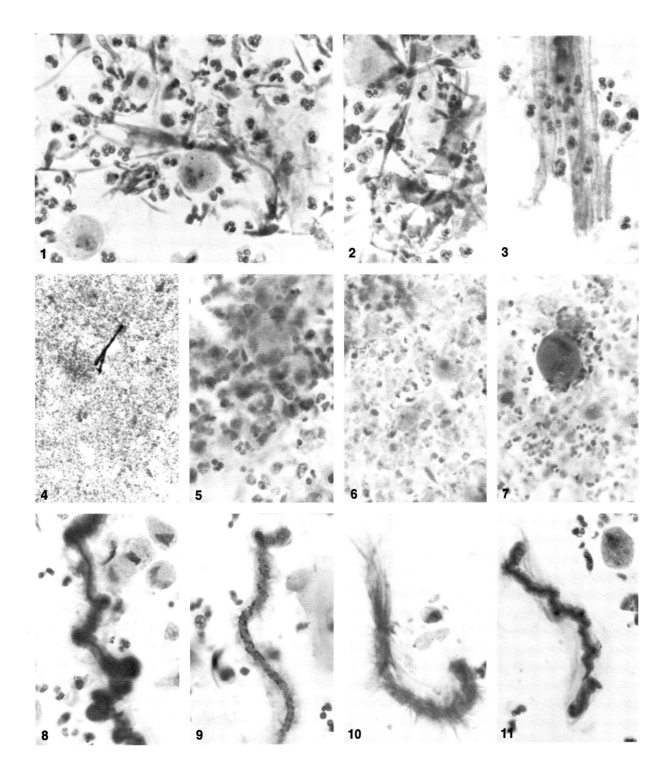

Plate 5

NORMAL BRONCHIAL EPITHELIAL LINING AND COLUMNAR CELLS IN SPUTUM

In Figure 1, the histological section of the bronchial lining is stained with hematoxylin-eosin and shows the tall columnar epithelial cells displaying the terminal eosinophilically stained bar (A) with the projecting cilia (B). The clear vacuoles of the goblet cells are almost equally spaced between the columnar cells. Usually, two to six layers of the nuclei are seen, in contrast to the many layers of the nuclei seen in sections of basal cell hyperplasia noted in Plate 10, Figure 2.

Figure 2 is a small cluster of tall columnar epithelium found in sputum revealing similar cellular detail as in Figure 1. Note the abundant cytoplasm in the luminal portion of these cells and their thin whip-like base.

Figure 3 shows numerous single, tall columnar cells. Some of the cells still show the terminal bars, while others are swollen and vacuolated with a cytoplasm in the process of degeneration and fragmentation. The large vacuolated cells may represent degenerating goblet cells, which do not show the terminal bar and cilia. It seems that the goblet cells fragment and degenerate much more rapidly than the tall columnar cells.

Figures 4–9 display clusters of tall columnar epithelial cells that show degeneration of most of the cytoplasm. The nuclei are well preserved although overlapping in some areas. The cuboidal arrangement of the cells, residual terminal bar, and cilia help identify these cells as degenerating columnar cells, rather than neoplastic cells. These figures show a progressive degree of degeneration, and it is interesting to note that the cilia disappear very early in this degeneration process.

Figures 10 and 11 reveal another variety of degenerating, tall, columnar epithelial cells. These show degeneration of the nuclei, which are black, markedly shrunken, with complete loss of nuclear particulate material. The cytoplasm is usually blue or blue-pink. The cells' residual elongation of cuboidal arrangement helps to identify them as being of tall columnar cell origin. Usually, these cells are seen in clusters but may be single and must be differentiated from metaplastic squamous cells.

REFERENCES

1. Auerbach O, et al: Changes in the bronchial epithelium in relation to smoking and cancer of the lung. N Engl J Med 256:97–104, 1957
2. Green GM: In defense of the lung. American Lung Association Bulletin 60: No. 3, April, 1974
3. Bloom W, Fawcett DW: A Textbook of Histology, ed 10. Philadelphia: W. B. Saunders Co., 1975

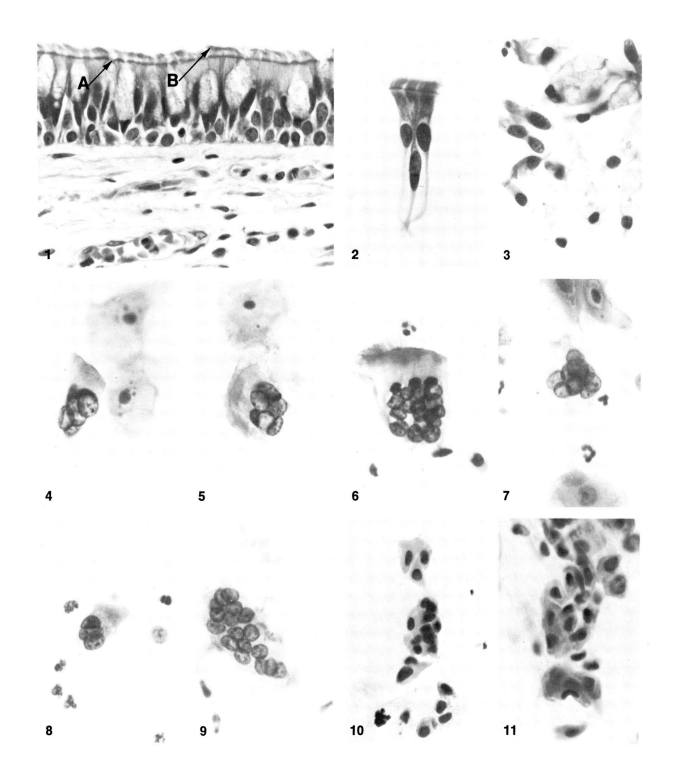

Plate 6

DEGENERATING COLUMNAR CELLS OF BRONCHIAL LINING ORIGIN

ABNORMAL COLUMNAR EPITHELIAL CELLS IN STAGES OF FRAGMENTATION AND DEGENERATION

The bronchial epithelium has a 30-day regeneration cycle and, as a result of this rapid cell turnover, many columnar cells are shed from the surface and discharged into the mucous blanket of the tracheobronchial tree. Many of these cells degenerate, fragment, and dissolve, while others survive to be found in expectorated bronchial exudate (sputum). A variety of cell forms in various phases of degeneration are found in the sputum samples. Some of these resemble tumor and may be pitfalls in diagnosis.[1]

Figures 1–4 are swollen nuclei with relatively coarse nuclear material, but the cytoplasm is retained along one border and shows cilia (Fig. 1) and a residual base or terminal bars (Figs. 2, 3, 4, 5, and 8), which aid in the identification of these cells as columnars. Figures 6, 7, 9, 10, 11, and 12 reveal coarse granular nuclear substance with some nuclear membrane folds, clefts and even areas of dissolution. The basophilic cytoplasm and its elongated arrangement always help to identify these cells as of columnar epithelial origin. As mentioned above and stressed here, these cells are frequently misinterpreted as malignant but are usually few in number or single, which aids in ruling out malignancy. It should be remembered that a diagnosis of malignancy should never be made from single or very few cells. In malignant cases, cells are usually shed, and therefore numerous tumor cells are revealed in the sputum sample.

Tumors that shed many malignant cells are WHO IB or IC (See Table 2, p 48), and the cells found in sputum from these tumors frequently simulate abnormal columnar cells. Cases showing these cell types are on Plates 23, 24, and 25. These cells, of course, should not be interpreted as abnormal columnars, but note some of the cell similarities.

REFERENCE

1. Koss LG, Richardson HL: Some pitfalls of cytological diagnosis of lung cancer. Cancer 8:937–947, 1955

22

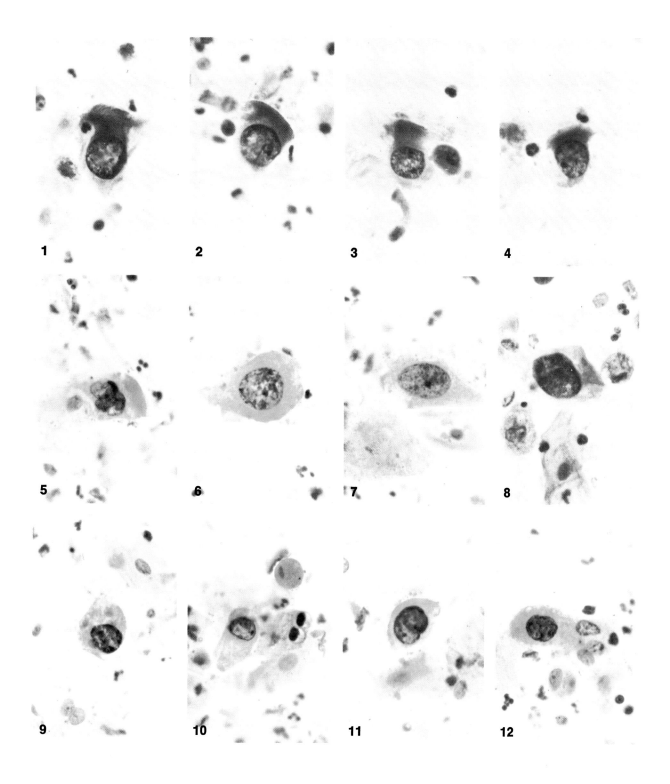

Plate 7

CELLS OF NASOPHARYNGEAL GLAND ORIGIN: A SPUTUM COMPONENT

The cells displayed in these photographs (Figs. 2, 3, 5, 6, 7, 8, 9, 10) are often seen admixed with cells of lung origin. It has been difficult to identify the exact origin of these cells, but their frequent observation in sputum from patients with upper respiratory viral or bacterial infections has led us to suspect that these cells arise in the upper respiratory tract. Sections of respiratory mucosa of the larynx, nasopharynx, and nasal cavity reveal cells in the mucosal glands that simulate the cells found in the exudates from these zones. Note the similarity of the cells that form the lining of the gland in Figure 1 with the cells seen in the lumen of this gland and their similarity to the cells seen in Figures 2 and 3, which are shown at a higher magnification. Also, note the cells lining the ducts of the glands seen in Figure 4 and those depicted in sputum samples in Figures 5–8. The nuclei are essentially of the same size, but may vary slightly. The cytoplasm is usually abundant and brightly orangeophilic. The cells in Figures 9 and 10 are from a nasal cytowash (cytogram) from a patient who had an upper respiratory viral infection. These cells simulate the cells described above. We have never seen malignancy in these cells. They are suspected of being of lung origin but, as mentioned above, originate primarily from upper respiratory infections. The origin of these cells suggested here deserves further investigation, since similar cells could originate in peribronchial glands. We feel that upper respiratory infections are probably the source of these cells, but, more importantly, they should be identified as benign.

24

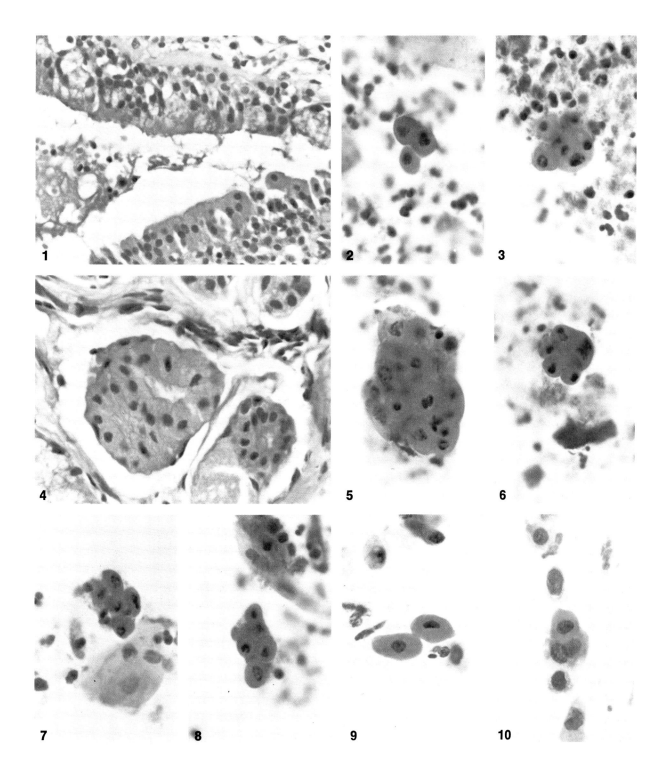

Plate 8

LÖFFLER'S SYNDROME: IDENTIFICATION BY SPUTUM CYTOLOGY

Löffler's syndrome is a pulmonary disease that is characterized by transitory, radiologically visible lung lesions, eosinophilia, and fever. Histologically, the pulmonary lesion (Fig. 1) shows alveolar exudate, alveolar cell proliferation, and inflammatory infiltrate, with an abundance of eosinophils. It has been suggested that the disease is an allergic reaction limited to the lung parenchyma, but may be related to other reticuloendothelial diseases. A mild productive cough, which is usually present in this affliction, affords an opportunity for cytological studies which can aid materially in confirming the diagnosis. The sputum cytological studies reveal clusters of epithelioid cells (Figs. 4–10) or single cells (Fig. 3) which may be of alveolar lining cell origin. The cells have regular nuclei with abundant bluish cytoplasm. The nuclear material is vesicular with prominent chromocenters. Eosinophils are numerous, and many large clusters of these cells are found (Fig. 2). The hyperchromatism of the epithelioid cells may elicit deep concern about malignancy, but the other benign features of the cells and the numerous eosinophils allay this concern. The disease responds very effectively to corticosteroid medication.

Abundant eosinophils are sometimes seen in the sputum of asthmatic patients. The epithelioid nests of cells, of course, are absent in these cases, and the clinical course is distinguished by the allergic picture usually confirmed by other clinical testing for allergies.

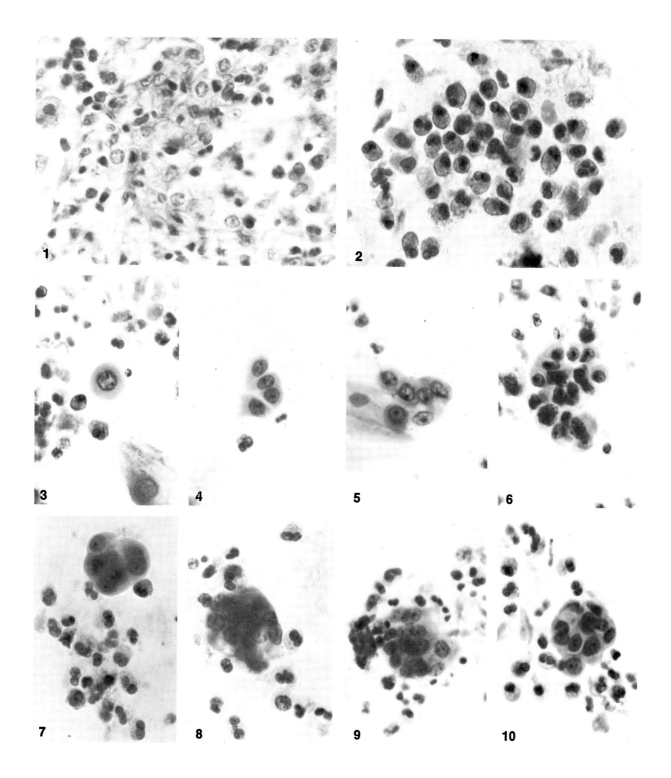

Plate 9

DEVELOPMENT OF CANCER OF THE LUNG

Plate 9 shows the various arbitrary stages of tumor development over a period of time from the normal lining of the lung to abnormal stages of squamous cell metaplasia. These changes ascend in atypia to develop into carcinoma in situ (CIS). This eventually develops into invasive cancer. This chart shows the development of epidermoid cancer, which takes about 10–15 years or more to develop. Other types of tumors of the lung that arise from the bronchial epithelium probably develop in this way, and the time period may be shorter. Further study is needed in these areas.

The chart is divided into three components, which depict the histology of this progression from left to right (upper row of photographs), starting with normal tall columnar epithelium, which ascends in degrees of atypia to malignancy. These histological sections show cell type and the relationships of cells to each other in the formation of the tissue. Study of these histological sections reveals a close relationship to the cells that are found in sputum (middle row of photographs), forming the next category. Note the similarity of the cells to the frame above. Study of the histological pattern in each frame with the cells depicted below will give a good understanding of the origin of the cells found in the sputum. This also reveals, for example, why cells in a mild atypical stage are frequently seen in clusters, since they peel off from the surface of the epithelium. Therefore they are seen as sheets of cells lying flat on the slide, while cells that are shed from the surface in moderate or marked atypia, or even in CIS are frequently seen as single cells because of the irregularity of the surface of these forms of epithelium. Information on cell size can be obtained by comparing the histology with the corresponding frames of cytology found in the sputum. Also note the degree of pleomorphism, staining intensity, etc.

In order to facilitate understanding of the various cell differences in these histological and cytological categories, the minute cell changes (criteria), as seen cytologically, are listed in each stage of atypia in Table 1. The sketches below the cytology are drawn from these criteria to emphasize the minute changes seen in each stage, presenting a methodological, point-by-point analysis for learning the histological and cytological features noted in each stage. A detailed understanding and review of the similarity of cells among the three rows of Plate 9 will help the student learn the basic features and aid in the cytological screening of pulmonary specimens.

28

DEVELOPMENT OF CARCINOMA OF THE LUNG

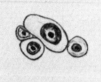

PHOTOMICROGRAPH OF HISTOLOGICAL SECTION

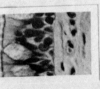

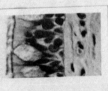
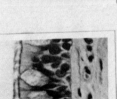
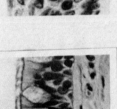
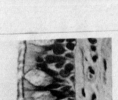

PHOTOMICROGRAPH OF SPUTUM CELLS

SKETCH

NORMAL	REGULAR	MILD	MODERATE	MARKED	CIS	INV. CA.
	SQUAMOUS	CELL	METAPLASIA			

The clinical significance of the cell patterns discussed above is poorly understood. Squamous cell metaplasia, particularly when atypical, can probably be explained by a carcinogenic effect and thus may be related to the development of neoplasia. Some writers question the development of carcinoma from squamous cell metaplasia, suggesting that it originates in the columnar epithelium.[1] Most authors, however, believe that the most likely source is squamous cell metaplasia,[2,3,4,5] since ascending atypias of metaplasia can be demonstrated to develop ultimately into carcinoma over a long period of time. If the latter is not true, there is a concomitant development or progression of atypical cells which accompany the tumor development.

REFERENCES

1. Melamed MR, et al: Radiologically occult in situ and incipient invasive epidermoid lung cancer. Am J Surg Pathol 1:5–16, 1977
2. Auerbach O, et al: Changes in the bronchial epithelium in relation to smoking and cancer of the lung. N Engl J Med 256:97–104, 1957
3. Nasiell M: Metaplasia and atypical metaplasia in the bronchial epithelium: A histopathologic and cytopathologic study. Acta Cytol 10:421–427, 1966
4. Papanicolaou GN: A survey of actualities and potentialities of exfoliative cytology in cancer diagnosis. Ann Intern Med 31:661–674, 1949
5. Saccomanno G, et al: Development of carcinoma of the lung as reflected in exfoliated cells. Cancer 33:256–270, 1974

TABLE 1 CYTOLOGICAL CRITERIA FOR SQUAMOUS CELL METAPLASIA AND EPIDERMOID CARCINOMA

Regular Metaplasia

1. Cells all of about same size.
2. Nuclei of same size with regular nuclear/cytoplasmic ratio.
3. Nuclear material fine and powdery with rare chromocenter.
4. Cytoplasm usually basophilic.
5. Cells usually occur in sheets, but may be single.

Metaplasia, Mild Atypia

1. Cells vary slightly in size.
2. Nuclei vary slightly in size, and nuclear/cytoplasmic ratio may vary slightly.
3. Nuclear material still fine and powdery with rare clusters of nuclear material near the nuclear membrane.
4. Cytoplasm may be acidophilic.
5. Cells usually occur in sheets, but may be found singly.

Metaplasia, Moderate Atypia

1. Cells vary moderately in size; some are smaller but most are larger than in mild metaplasia.
2. Nuclei vary significantly in size with moderate variation in nuclear/cytoplasmic ratio.
3. Nuclear material is still fine and powdery in most areas, but nuclear masses are abundant, particularly along the membrane.
4. Nuclear lobulations, crevices, and nodules are present.
5. Cytoplasm may be basophilic, but acidophilia predominates.
6. Cells usually occur in sheets, but an increase in singles is found.

Metaplasia, Marked Atypia

1. Cells vary markedly in size, but are generally larger than the moderate atypias.
2. Nuclear pleomorphism is marked, and nuclear material is coarse and sometimes clustered about the nuclear membrane. Nuclear/cytoplasmic ratio varies, with extremes.
3. Nucleoli are present but are small and may be acidophilic.
4. Acidophilic cytoplasm predominates.
5. Single cells predominate.

Carcinoma in situ

1. Cells vary in size and may be double the size of marked metaplasia. Single cells are present, but clusters are more common than in invasive carcinoma.
2. The nuclear material is coarse and accumulates in large masses, but the concentrations are not usually accumulated near the membrane. Chromocenters are large and simulate nucleoli, but are not always acidophilic.
3. The nuclear/cytoplasmic ratio is decreased in some, while increased in others, causing obvious nuclear pleomorphism.
4. Cannibalism and multinucleation may be present.
5. Acidophilic cytoplasm predominates.

Invasive Carcinoma

1. Cells are larger, but may be very pleomorphic and bizarre. They usually are single, but clusters are found.
2. Nuclear material is coarse and accumulates in masses unevenly around the nuclear membrane.
3. Nucleoli are large and acidophilic.
4. Increased and decreased nuclear/cytoplasmic ratio.
5. Cannibalism and multinucleation are common.
6. Cytoplasm is acidophilic and basophilic.

(From Saccomanno.[5] Used with permission.)

Plate 10

VARIETIES OF BRONCHIAL EPITHELIUM

The varieties of bronchial epithelium shown in Plate 10 are the following: Figure 1, normal; Figure 2, basal cell hyperplasia; Figures 3 – 6, varieties of squamous cell metaplasia; and Figure 7, metaplasia of infarct.

The carcinogenic effect on the tracheobronchial tree has received much attention in the last 30 years. Auerbach[1,2] (personal communication, 1969), in a detailed analysis of a large population of cigarette smokers and nonsmokers noted that a variety of epithelial changes occurred in those exposed patients. These changes are shown here to give the student of cytology some understanding of the histological patterns of the development of the cells found in sputum. Figure 1, here and on Plate 5, shows normal, tall columnar epithelium of the upper and lower respiratory tract. Obviously, the only cells shed from this epithelium would be either of the tall ciliated cell type or of the goblet cell variety that do not show the terminal eosinophilic bar or the cilia. Note that some of the cells just above the basement membrane appear not to reach the surface. These have been called reserve or basal cells and have been assumed to be the generative cells from which the ciliated or goblet cells originate. Possibly, these cells may give rise to basal cell hyperplasia (Fig. 2) or to tumors of the respiratory tract.[3] Others feel that the origin of squamous cell carcinoma is from metaplastic squamous epithelium.[4] Figure 2 shows a very common variety of basal cell hyperplasia. Patients who have been exposed to respiratory carcinogens nearly always show this type of hyperplasia. It is found most abundantly in the primary bronchi but is also seen in secondary bronchioles or even more peripherally. When Figure 2 is compared to Figure 1, both with the same magnification, one notes, in the former, the increased thickness and many layers of nuclei. Some of the cells reach the surface of the epithelium and have terminal bars and cilia. Goblet cells are still present, but the goblets are smaller and fewer in number. The epithelium shown in Figure 1 would shed normal cells, and that in Figure 2 would shed cells that are indistinguishable from normal because both are tall columnar cells. Figure 3 shows a slightly more advanced hyperplasia with some transition to squamous metaplasia. Terminal bars are not present and cilia are conspicuously absent. In fact, the superficial layers are squamoid, but the polarity of the deeper cells is still similar to the hyperplasia. Figure 3 would shed cells of a regular metaplastic cell type, showing no atypia.

Figures 4, 5, and 6 show three other varieties of squamous cell metaplasia that are less common but may be found in bronchi of all sizes. There is considerable evidence that the squamoid tumors of the respiratory tree arise from metaplasia which, cytologically, can be categorized into mild, moderate, and marked atypias. These squamous cell metaplasias, along with the basal cell hyperplasia, are frequently seen to adjoin carcinoma in situ.

Over a relatively long period of time (3 – 15 years), these cells can be demonstrated to become progressively more and more atypical and eventually to de-

33

velop into carcinoma. Many of these atypical squamous metaplastic cells have been demonstrated in cases in which polyploidal neoplasia developed long before the cells became sufficiently atypical to be placed in the category of marked atypia.[5]

Figure 7 shows an area of squamous cell metaplasia found in the lung of a patient who had repeated bouts of pulmonary embolism with infarct. Some of the infarcts did not resolve, and one was removed surgically because it was suspected of being malignant. The cells shown here were embedded in organized scar tissue. The pleomorphism of these cells suggests that this may explain the origin of squamous cell carcinoma in peripheral scars. Cells from an area of this type probably could not reach the bronchial tree, and this may be a reasonable explanation for the low yield of tumor cells from peripheral scar lesions of the lung.

Most writers support the thesis that the epidermoid tumors, including the adenosquamous cell carcinoma, develop from squamous cell metaplasia (see Plate 26).

REFERENCES

1. Auerbach O, et al: Smoking habits and age in relation to pulmonary changes; rupture of alveolar septums, fibrosis and thickening of walls of small arteries and arterioles. N Engl J Med. 269:1045–1054, 1963
2. Auerbach O, et al: Changes in bronchial epithelium in relation to cigarette smoking and in relation to lung cancer. N Engl J Med 265:253–267, 1961
3. Melamed MR, et al: Radiologically occult in situ and incipent invasive epidermoid lung cancer. Am J Surg Pathol 1:5–16, 1977
4. Saccomanno G, et al: Development of carcinoma of the lung as reflected in exfoliated cells. Cancer 33:256–270, 1974
5. Nasiell M, et al: Cytomorphological grading and Fuelgen DNA-analysis of metaplastic and neoplastic bronchial cells. Cancer 41:1511–1521, 1978

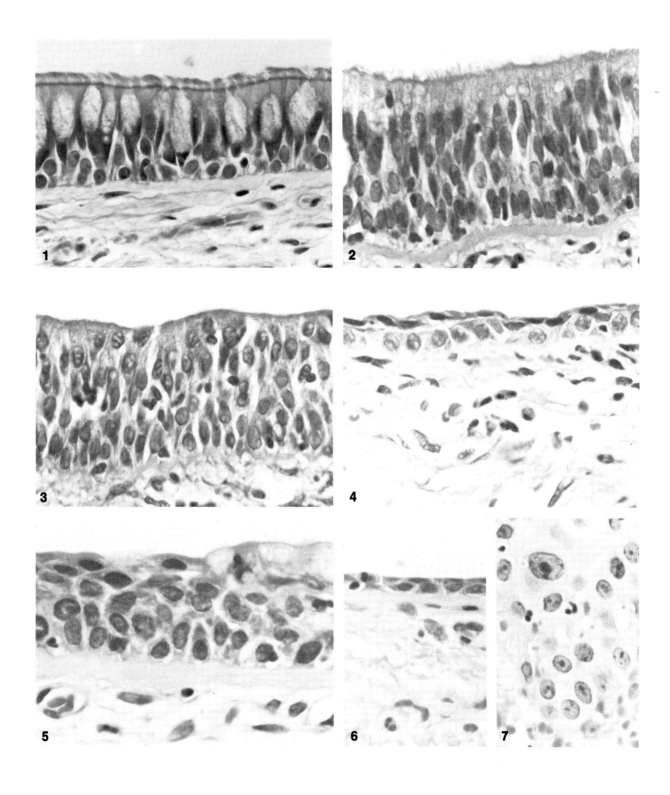

Plate 11

REGULAR SQUAMOUS CELL METAPLASIA

Figure 1 is a section of bronchus showing regular squamous cell metaplasia. Figures 2–11 show sheets of cells found in sputum samples. Note the regular nuclear/cytoplasmic ratio and the fine granular, nuclear material. These cells, even when in clusters or sheets, lie flat on the slide, and all the cells are in focus. This suggests that they peel off from the surface of the metaplastic layer. This type of squamous cell metaplasia is very common in sections of the bronchial tree, and we suspect that similar cells may arise from the alveolar lining cells. Frequently, this type of metaplasia may alternate with and adjoin zones of basal cell hyperplasia. The thickness of this type of metaplasia is usually as shown here, showing 8 to 15 layers of cells, but sometimes it is only two to three layers thick. Once in a while it may be seen as only one layer of cells.

The cause of regular squamous cell metaplasia may be due to chronic inflammation, infarct (Plate 10, Fig. 7), or to carcinogenic effect. Of course, it may also be due to vitamin A deficiency. Approximately 7–11% of the patients who are seen in a physician's office or are admitted to the hospital because of pulmonary pathology will have regular squamous cell metaplasia. Moreover, all cases showing a more severe type of atypia will also have regular metaplasia.[1]

REFERENCES

1. Saccomanno G: Atypical metaplasia of the bronchial epithelium; frequency and significance, a preliminary report. (Unpublished)

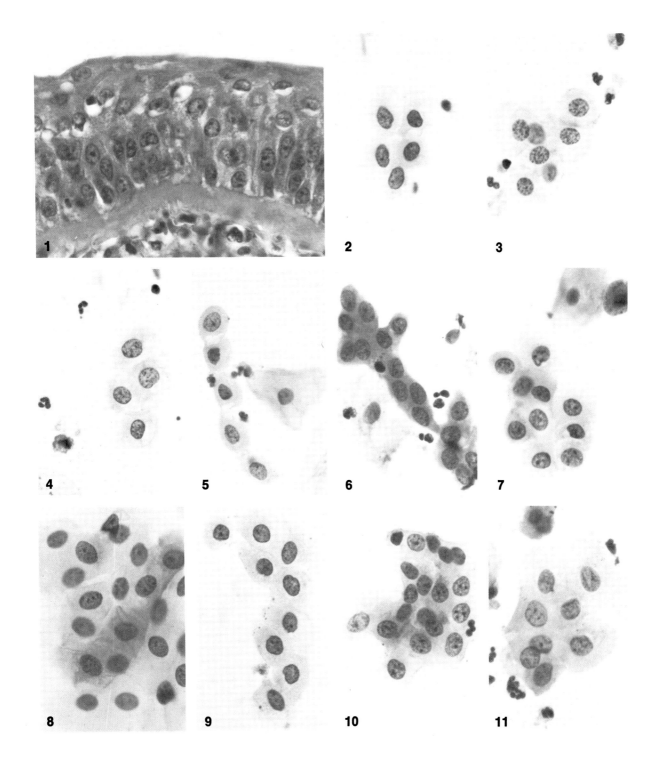

Plate 12

MILD ATYPICAL SQUAMOUS CELL METAPLASIA

Figure 1 is a histological section of a secondary bronchus with a mild atypical squamous cell metaplasia, showing a minimal degree of pleomorphism and minimal hyperchromasia. This type of squamous cell metaplasia is the most common type of atypia seen in the bronchial tree[1] (see Table 1, p 31). The epithelium varies in thickness, depending on how much stretching occurred as a result of fixation with fluid. It is sometimes seen as a thick layer, even when there has been no stretching due to fixation. Thicker epithelium (many layers of cells) may suggest that dilating the tracheobronchial tree does not have any effect on the lining. Mild atypical squamous cell metaplasia is so frequently seen cytologically in sputum that it is thought to be a response to infection of the tracheobronchial tree.

Figures 2–11 display cells in sputum showing mild atypia. These cells are generally smaller than regular squamous metaplastic cells and usually are seen in adhesive clusters. They lie flat and apparently represent sheets of cells which have peeled off from underlying, less mature cells. Some of the cells in these clusters are eosinophilically stained, while others are basophilic. The significance of this is not completely understood. The nuclear material of these cells is still finely granular or vesicular, and occasional chromocenters are noted. The nuclear/cytoplasmic ratio is slightly increased in some cells. Since these cells lie flat on the slide, all of the nuclei are in focus, as is the cytoplasm.

REFERENCE

1. Saccomanno G, et al: Development of carcinoma of the lung as reflected in exfoliated cells. Cancer 33:256–270, 1974

38

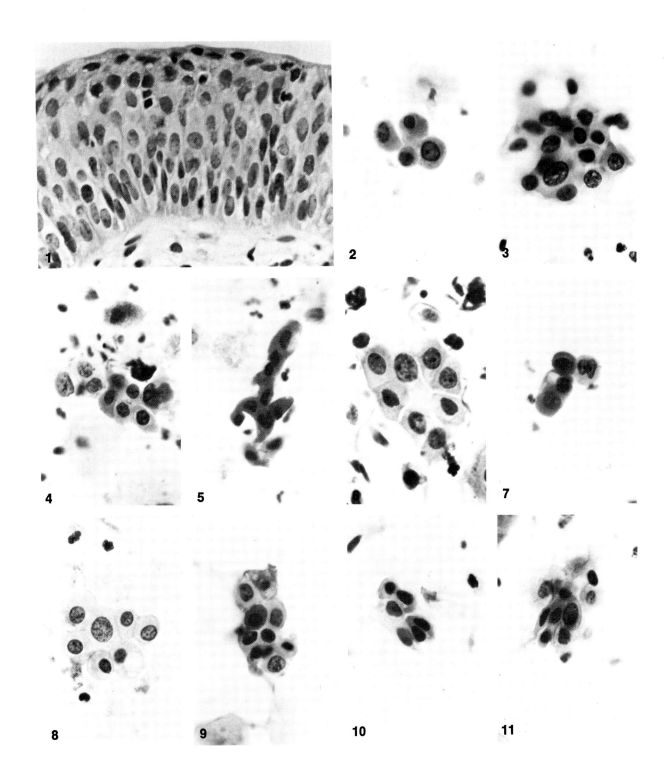

Plate 13

FIBER CELLS IN MILD ATYPICAL SQUAMOUS CELL METAPLASIA

Figure 1 is an area of bronchus that reveals a mild squamous cell metaplasia with flattened cells on the surface showing fiber cell formation. Fiber cells tend to be elongated, and the cytoplasm appears to be stretched along a longitudinal axis resulting in cells that frequently are more than 200–300 μ in length. These cells vary in width because they are spindle-shaped but in the central area measure 20–30 μ in width. The origin of the cells shown here is the surface of a mild squamous cell metaplasia, but they are often seen in the layer nearest the lumen in metaplasia of two or three cell layers. Mild atypical squamous cell metaplasia is seen cytologically so frequently in sputum that it is thought to be a response to infection of the tracheobronchial tree.

The nuclei are usually elongated, have a distinct nuclear membrane, and are composed of a fine reticular to granular matrix. The cytoplasm is usually yellow-orange and bright. Frequently, the cells are single (Figs. 2–4) but may be in clusters (Figs. 5, 6). These cells are keratinizing and sometimes form whorls around a central core of keratin to form epithelial pearls. It is important to distinguish these benign cells from the malignant fibers seen in keratinizing squamous cell carcinoma (see Plate 21).

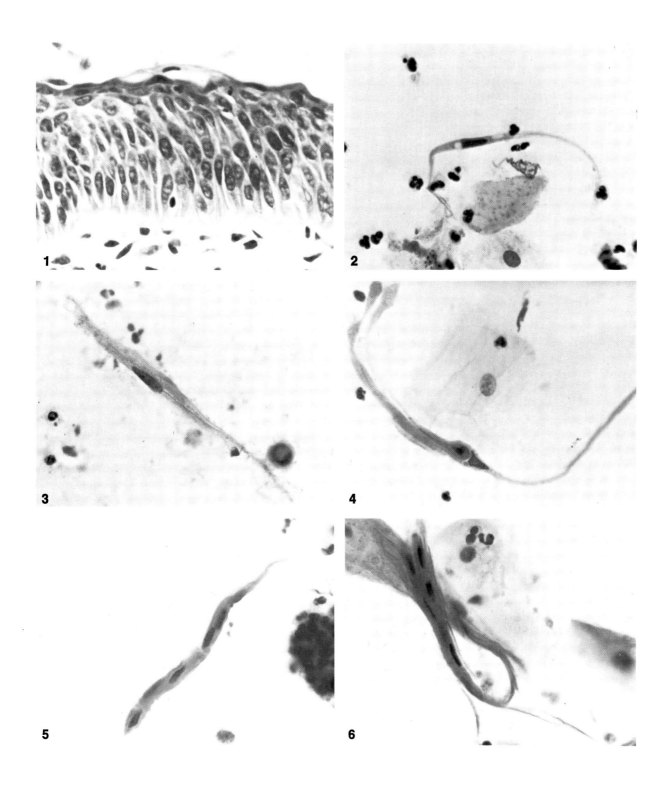

Plate 14

MODERATE ATYPICAL SQUAMOUS CELL METAPLASIA

Figure 1 is a histological section of a secondary bronchus showing moderate, atypical, squamous cell metaplasia. This section is of about average thickness, but much thicker zones are noted occasionally, and still other areas are thinner. Generally, the moderate, atypical, squamous pattern shows some distortion of cell polarity, and the section appears more deeply stained with basic stains. The nuclear pleomorphism is very distinct, and the epithelial layers often rest on a thickened, hyaline, basement membrane. Frequently, one will observe lymphocytic infiltration beneath the basement membrane, which is present to a minimal degree in this section.

Figures 2–22 show moderate, atypical metaplastic squamous cells found in sputum. These cells may still peel off from the underlying epithelium and are often found in sheets, as seen in Figures 2, 6, 7, 8, 9, and 10. Generally, these cells are slightly larger than mild atypical cells. They flatten out on the slide, and the nuclear/cytoplasmic ratio is easily evaluated because of this flattening. These are seen as single cells more frequently than those in mild atypia. The nuclei vary significantly in size, and some stain deeply basophilic (Figs. 2, 3, 6, 7, 9, 10), while others stain eosinophilically to bright yellow. The nuclear material appears abundant and coarse in some cells, while in others it accumulates along the nuclear membrane. The membrane is smooth. Many of these cells with large nuclei and abundant nuclear material may have increased DNA.[1]

These cells are worrisome since, in many instances, they have been the precursors to more advanced atypias and malignancy. Further observations are needed to assess incidence and reversibility of these cell changes if carcinogens are removed.

REFERENCE

1. Nasiell M, et al: Cytomorphological grading and Feulgen DNA-analysis of metaplastic and neoplastic bronchial cells. Cancer 41:1511–1521, 1978

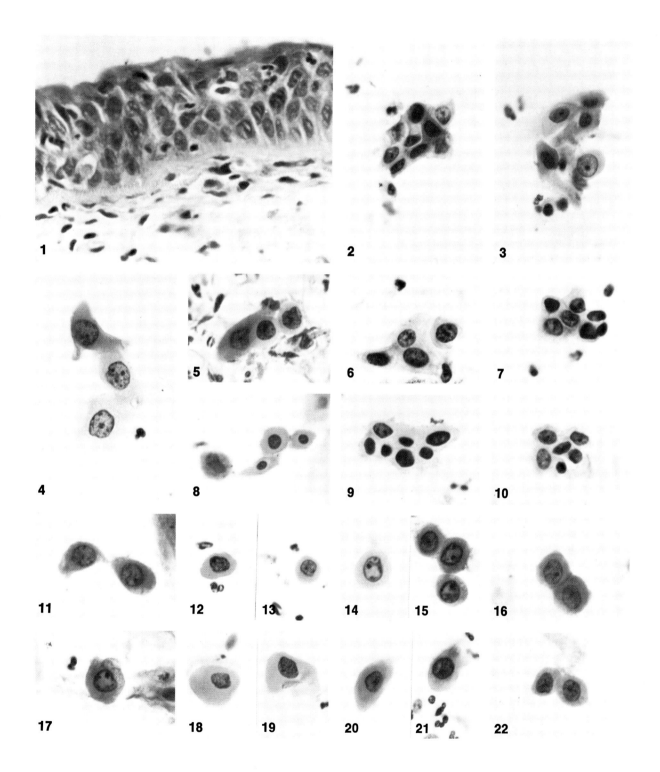

1

2

3

4

5

6

7

8

9

10

11

12

13

14

15

16

17

18

19

20

21

22

Plate 15

MARKED ATYPICAL SQUAMOUS CELL METAPLASIA

Figure 1 is a section of a secondary bronchus that shows one variety of marked atypical squamous cell metaplasia. Sometimes this stage of atypia is much thicker, showing many cell layers (up to 30), while in other areas it may be much thinner (one to two cell layers). The cellular arrangement reveals some loss of polarity, nuclear pleomorphism, and varied nuclear/cytoplasmic ratios. The epithelial cell layers at the surface show some atypical fiber-cell formation with deeply stained basophilic nuclei. In fact, the nuclei are shrunken, hardly showing nuclear detail. This type of epithelium is again seen to cover a thickened basement membrane.

Figures 2–21 show a variety of cells which exhibit the many characteristics of marked atypia. These cells vary markedly in size, with some measuring 70–90 μ in length (Fig. 10), and others (Figs. 18, 19), 10–15 μ in diameter. The nuclear/cytoplasmic ratio is varied, and the nuclear material is coarse (Figs. 5, 10, 11, 14, 16). These cells are worrisome and, when seen, deserve continued search in order to be positive that one is dealing with atypia rather than carcinoma in situ. When stained with Feulgen fluorescent stain, many of these cells show increased DNA, indicating bizarre chromosomal products frequently seen in malignancy. The great majority of patients showing this cytological atypia will ultimately develop neoplasia;[1,2] such patients should be followed with frequent sputum cytology in order to identify, as soon as possible, the malignant cells that will eventually appear, so that localization of the lesion can be made. If fiberoptic bronchoscopy or cytology fails to identify the malignant lesion at an early stage of development, frequent chest X-rays should be done in order to identify the lesion as early as possible.

REFERENCES

1. Nasiell M, et al: Cytomorphological grading and Feulgen DNA-Analysis of metaplastic and neoplastic bronchial cells. Cancer 41:1511–1521, 1978
2. Kato H, et al: Cytophotometric DNA analysis in atypical squamous metaplasia of bronchial epithelium. Outline of Principal Research Projects, Department of Surgery, Tokyo Medical College, October, 1976

44

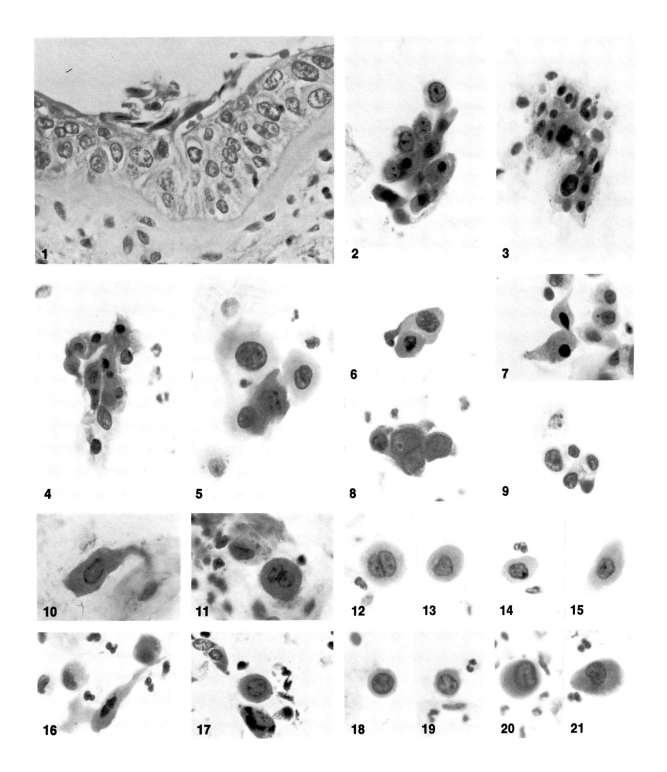

Plate 16

CARCINOMA IN SITU (CIS)

Figure 1 is a section of a lesion in situ. The thickness seen in the figure is usual for carcinoma in situ. The cell arrangement shows minimal squamoid polarity and many of the cells display marked nuclear pleomorphism with hyperchromasia. No invasion is noted. The cytology of CIS is usually in the form of single cells. Rare syncytia or paired cells are found. The cells of keratinizing epidermoid tumors are rather large, with many reaching 100 μ or more in diameter. Sometimes the cytoplasm is well preserved and orangeophilic, as is noted in Figures 3 and 7–9, but it may also be basophilic (Figs. 2, 9, 10, 11). Occasionally, only ghost remains of the cytoplasm are noted (Figs. 6, 11). Lobulations of the nuclei are frequently seen in both invasive and noninvasive keratinizing epidermoid lesions, and occasionally cannibalism is noted (Fig. 8). The nuclear material is usually visible, coarse, and often interrupted by clear zones, and these features always play a large role in the diagnosis of malignancy. The nuclear membrane is usually intact but may show interruptions or breaks, such as mouse bites, depressions, crevices, sharp angulations, and thickened areas, which are difficult to separate from large accumulations of nuclear substances or masses.

REFERENCES

1. Sanderson DR, Fontana RS: Early lung cancer detection and localization. Ann Otol Rhinol Laryngol 84:583–588, 1975
2. Woolner LB, Andersen HA, Bernatz PE: Occult carcinoma of the bronchus: A study of 15 cases in situ or early invasive bronchogenic carcinoma. Dis Chest 37:278–288, 1960
3. Woolner LB, et al: In situ and early invasive bronchogenic carcinoma. J Thorac Cardiovasc Surg 60:275–290, 1970

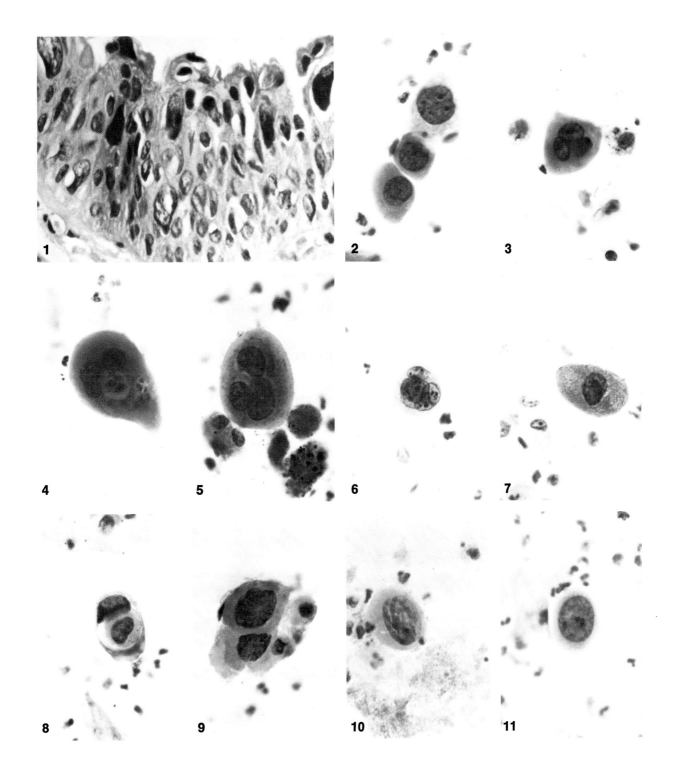

Plate 17
NUCLEAR DEBRIS

This case is presented to demonstrate one of the origins of nuclear debris in sputum samples. This case was of a 51-year-old female who had smoked cigarettes for about 20 years. She had been seen and treated for bronchitis, acute and chronic. Sputum studies were not done at this time, but X-ray films were negative. One year later, she was seen again with abdominal symptoms, and the chest X-ray at this time revealed a small mass in the right upper lobe of the lung. Induced sputum revealed tumor cells which are described below. A right upper lobectomy was performed following mediastinoscopy.

Sections of the tumor (Figs. 1–4) reveal epidermoid carcinoma (WHO IA, Table 2) showing numerous zones of necrosis surrounded by very actively growing tumor. The features of the sputum samples (Figs. 5–9) reveal similar qualities, consisting of abundant tumor tissue in varying degrees of degeneration. In one of the sections (Fig. 4), hardly any recognizable tumor cells are found, and the sputum smear (Fig. 8) shows a similar degree of degenerative diathesis. Another section (Fig. 2) and some of the smears (Figs. 7, 8) show cells which are less degenerated and preserved sufficiently well to at least suggest tumor. Finally, Figure 9 reveals two well-preserved cells that have all of the characteristics of neoplasia. Assessing all of these qualities of the sputum samples allows one to make a positive diagnosis of malignancy. Whenever sputum samples reveal abundant nuclear debris, one should suspect neoplasia, even though a definitive diagnosis cannot be made. Usually, additional sputum studies will yield cells sufficiently well preserved to establish a positive diagnosis.

Tumor degeneration is not the only cause of degenerated cellular elements in sputum positive for tumor, but it may well be a major one. Other causes are poor preservation, or possibly the position of the primary tumor which, if peripheral, may yield cells which degenerate before reaching the sputum cup.

TABLE 2 WORLD HEALTH ORGANIZATION
HISTOPATHOLOGICAL CLASSIFICATION OF LUNG TUMORS*

I. Epidermoid carcinoma
   A. Squamous cells with pearls, intercellular bridges, and keratin
   B. Squamous cells with intercellular bridges
   C. Sheets of slightly undifferentiated cells
II. Small cell, anaplastic carcinoma
   A. Small cell, lymphocyte-like (oat cell)
   B. Undifferentiated large polygonal, with sheets
III. Adenocarcinomas
   A. Bronchogenic
      1. Acinar
      2. Papillary
   B. Bronchiolo-alveolar
IV. Large cell carcinoma
   A. Solid tumors with or without mucus
   B. Giant and clear cell carcinomas
V. Adenosquamous carcinoma
VI. Carcinoid tumors
VII. Bronchial gland tumors
   A. Cylindromas
   B. Muco-epidermoid
VIII. Others
   A. Papillary tumors
   B. Mixed carcinosarcomas
   C. Sarcomas
   D. Mesotheliomas
   E. Melanomas

*Oslo, Norway, 1948; modified version.
NOTE: The World Health Organization Histopathological Classification of Lung Tumors published in 1967 was revised in October of 1977 in Geneva under the Chairmanship of Raymond Yesner, MD. This revision is expected to be published in 1979 and will not alter the basic classification of the major groups of lung carcinomas as referred to in this text.

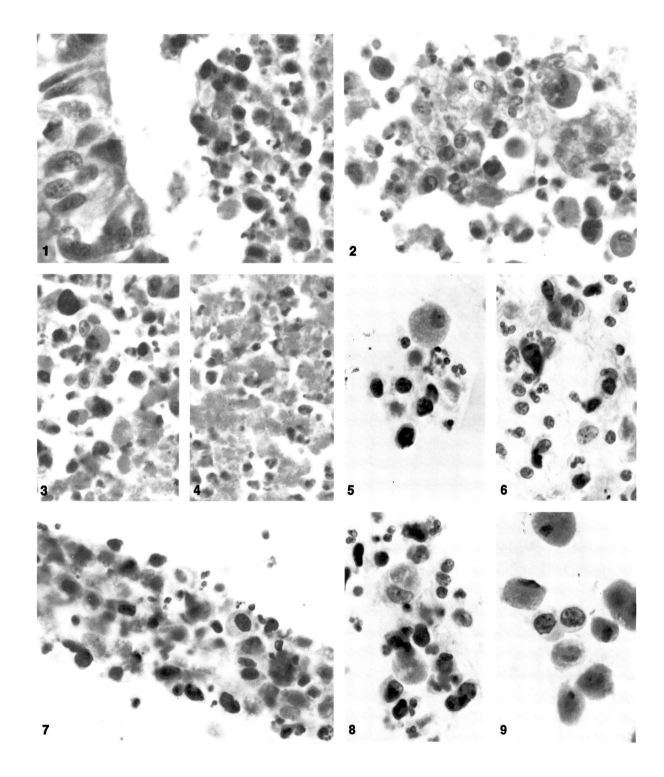

Plate 18

CARCINOMA, SQUAMOUS (WHO IA)

This plate reveals a variety of malignant cells from a 70-year-old patient with keratinizing epidermoid carcinoma (WHO IA). This is the most common tumor of the lung in man. The figures in this plate show only a small portion of the cells seen in this case. Although some of the cells seen here measure more than 125 μ in length (Figs. 10 and 11), other cells not photographed were even larger. Many of the cells, particularly those in Figures 1, 3, 6, 8, 9, 10, and 11, are classical keratinizing orangeophilic cells, while those in Figures 2, 5, 7, 12, and 16 are basophilic. It is still not known which type of cell grows more rapidly and which type predominates in the tumor after it has multiplied extensively and is seen on section. Generally, the less keratinized cells are more frequently seen in the premalignant and early malignant phase of tumorigenesis. The final cytological features of a tumor used in determining the WHO classification may have, however, very little resemblance to the cells seen in the sputum samples for several years during development of the tumor.

Another interesting feature of this case is the size of the basophilically stained cells. Some of the cells are very large (Figs. 2, 12) while others (Figs. 13, 14, 15) are small, the range being 30–120 μ. In spite of the variation among these tumor cells, one still notes that all belong to the same family, giving this tumor a unique personality.

It is usually not difficult to diagnose a case of this type when so many cells with such a wide variety of anaplastic features are present. It must be remembered, however, that at times only the small cells are shed from the tumor surface and are available for interpretation in the sputum sample. This case indicates that when the patient has a malignancy, the lesion sheds an abundance of cells. We have noted that when tumors are so small that they cannot be seen on X-ray or even on fiberoptic bronchoscopy, they still shed an abundance of cells. All of this supports the thesis that patients who have a malignancy, regardless of how small, still have many cells in their sputum. When single cells considered suspicious of malignancy are found, these are often artifacts, degenerating columnars, or some other pitfall. Thus the axiom—never make a diagnosis of malignancy on the basis of one suspicious cell—is important.

50

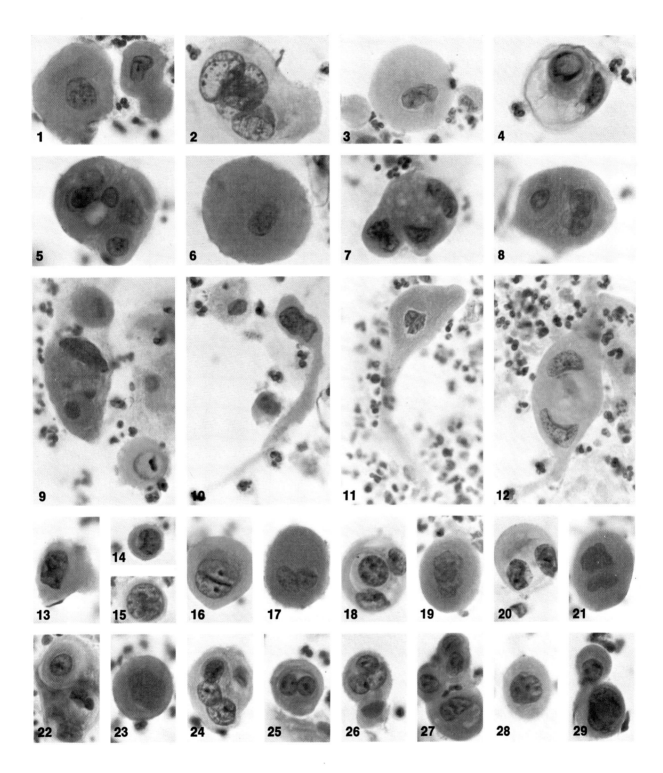

Plate 19

CARCINOMA, SQUAMOUS (WHO IA)

Figure 1 is another section of an invasive squamous cell carcinoma (WHO IA) from a 39-year-old male cigarette smoker for 15 years and uranium miner for 15 years. Tumors such as this are readily recognized with a high degree of accuracy.[1] The bizarre shape, orangeophilia, and nuclear pleomorphism of the cells facilitate diagnosis of these lesions in sputum smears. Sputum cytological examination results in a positive diagnosis in about 70–80% of these lesions seen on X-ray. If sputum examination is done frequently on susceptible high-risk patients, a much higher percentage (85–90%) can be identified. The cells reveal marked pleomorphism (Figs. 2, 4, 7) usually not seen in similar tumors in the carcinoma-in-situ stage, and many of the tumor cells have prominent acidophilic nucleoli which are abundant in the invasive lesions. Some cells have keratin and form epithelial pearls (Figs. 2, 4). Many of the cells are unusually large, form fibers (not shown here), or may be in clusters producing abundant orangeophilic keratin. Syncytia are seen (Fig. 2), but single cells are more common. The nuclei of these tumors have very coarse substance with large accumulations along the membrane. Clear areas are noted in the nuclei (Figs. 1, 3, 4, 5, 6, 7, 8). Nuclear pleomorphism is obvious, and the cytoplasm is abundant, but some cells have a marked increase in the nuclear/cytoplasmic ratio. Incidentally, this case revealed progressive atypical cell changes, and when the tumor developed, it was localized and removed, with no recurrences after six years. The patient has quit smoking and mining, and his sputum cytology reveals a mild, atypical squamous cell metaplasia.

Other cases of tumors in the squamous cell tumor group (WHO I) will be presented in the following plates to show the varied histological and cytological patterns among these lesions.

REFERENCE

1. Yesner R: Observer variability and reliability in lung cancer diagnosis. Cancer Chemother Rep 4:55–57, 1973

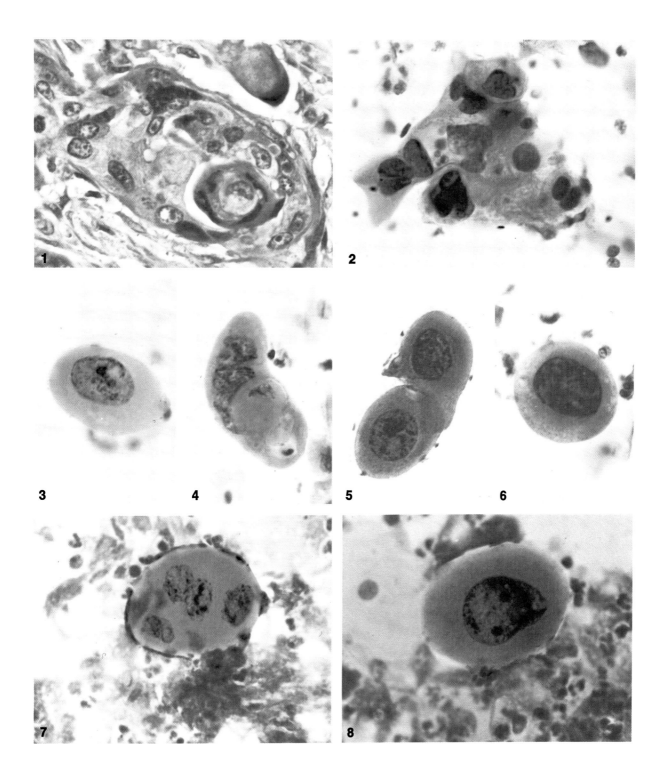

Plate 20

CARCINOMA, SQUAMOUS (WHO IA)

This case is of a 66-year-old tungsten miner who was also a heavy cigarette smoker for many years. The first cellular changes noted in his sputum at age 56 (Fig. 1) were called mild atypical squamous cell metaplasia. Three years later, his cells revealed moderate atypia (Fig. 2), and eight months later cells considered suspicious of carcinoma (Fig. 3) were found. A year later (Fig. 4) cells identified as positive for carcinoma were found, and the same result was obtained nine months after that (Fig. 5). X-rays of the chest were negative. Fiberoptic bronchoscopy yielded the cells from the left upper lobe (Fig. 6), which were called positive for invasive squamous cell carcinoma. The left upper lobe was resected (Fig. 7). No evidence of lymph node involvement was found, and Figure 8 reveals a section of the tumor shown in Figure 7. The patient made an uneventful recovery, and a year later, his sputum revealed mild atypia (Fig. 9). Figures 10 and 11 are cells found, respectively, in the first and second years following the resection and were diagnosed as positive for carcinoma in situ.

This is a classical case of squamous cell carcinoma with the probable development of a second tumor rather than a recurrence. This occurs in 22% of epidermoid carcinoma removals. Obviously, however, the tumor would probably have grown rapidly if it had not been removed. Probably, the second tumor will take an additional four or five years before it will become a serious problem, which indicates that, although a patient may have a second tumor, the survival period justifies the removal of the first lesion.

The cytology of the second tumor (Figs. 10, 11) is similar to that of the first lesion, and the prominent nucleoli suggest that this lesion is invasive. The patient's chest X-ray, however, is still negative. Characteristically, these lesions show prominent acidophilic nucleoli as is seen in Figures 5, 6, 8, 9, and 10. This feature usually indicates invasive carcinoma as is shown in Figures 6 and 8.

Figure 7 also reveals prominent emphysematous blebs in the lower portion of the photograph. This is a very common observation in patients who have had a long history of cigarette smoking. In some cases, this disease is so advanced that the patient does not have adequate pulmonary functional reserves, and this prevents surgical excision of the tumor.

REFERENCE

1. Ioachim HL: Progress in lung cancer. New York: Columbia University. (Unpublished)

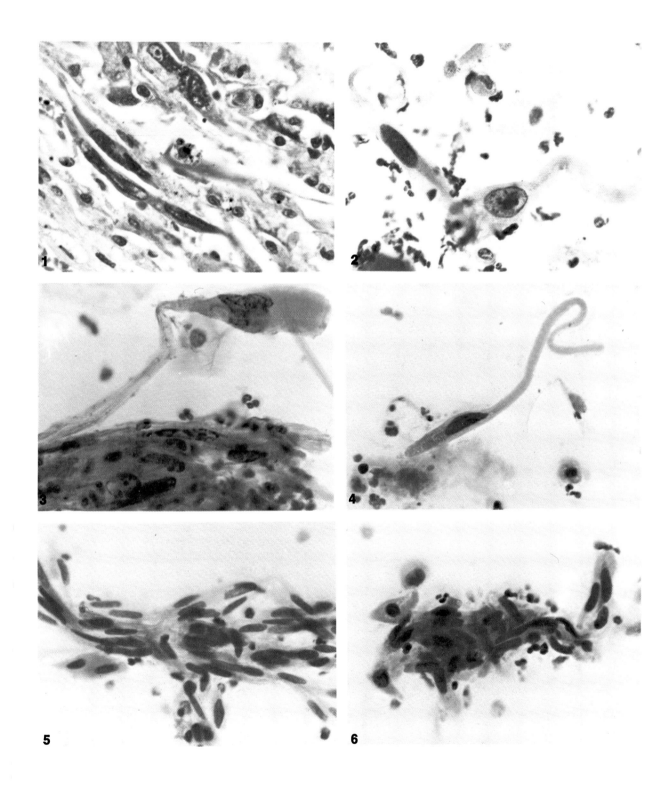

Plate 22

DEVELOPMENT OF CARCINOMA, SQUAMOUS (WHO IB)

This series of sputum samples (Figs. 1–10) reveals a progression of cellular changes beginning, in this male at age 53, as regular metaplastic squamous cells (Fig. 1). Figure 2 shows a nest of cells that were noted two years later. These cells have pleomorphic nuclei with fine granular chromatin, showing mild to moderate atypia. Figure 3 reveals a nest of cells, some of which are basophilically stained, while one is orangeophilic. The cells are disorganized, but the nuclei are more uniform than those in Figure 2, still revealing some pleomorphism. Figure 4 is worrisome because this cell has marked degeneration of the cytoplasm. The nucleus contains coarse nuclear material with some clear areas and shows a moderate degree of atypia. The cells in Figures 5, 6, 7, and 8 are all large orangeophilic cells showing progressively coarser nuclear material. The cells in Figures 6, 7, and 8 have sufficient nuclear change for one to suspect early malignant change. Figures 9 and 10 are of smaller cells with increased nuclear/cytoplasmic ratios. The cell in Figure 9 has coarse nuclear material with some clearing areas of the nucleus and what appears to be an acidophilic nucleolus. Figures 3–7 are pictures taken three years after the initial changes and two years prior to the invasive carcinoma seen in Figure 11, which has a variety of cells and is classed as a squamous cell carcinoma (WHO IB). This case took about five years to develop from a benign cytology to invasive carcinoma, and the invasive area was very small (micro-invasion).

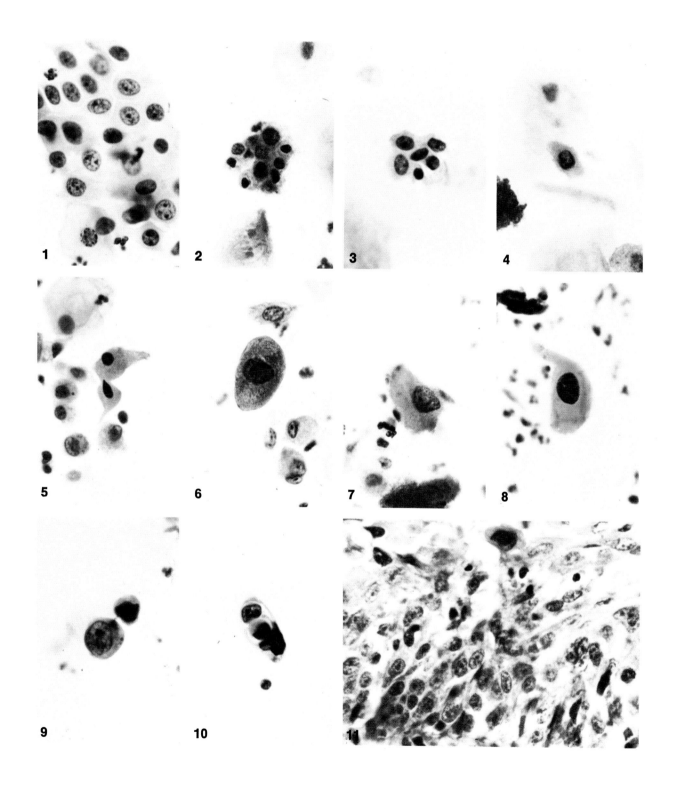

Plate 23

CARCINOMA, SQUAMOUS (WHO IB)

This case is of an 88-year-old male sheepherder with an unknown smoking history. This patient had a tumor (WHO IB) that shed a variety of cells that were rather uniform in size and had a very high nuclear/cytoplasmic ratio. It is important to note that these tumor cells are rather small, 25–30 μ in diameter, when compared to keratinizing cells which are frequently over 100 μ in diameter and may be much larger. This feature often results in a false negative diagnosis or an erroneous diagnosis of lymphoma, since these cells do simulate large lymphocytes having a relatively marked increase in nuclear/cytoplasmic ratio. If one is considering a diagnosis of lymphoma, this is dispelled by noting that these cells are almost twice the size of lymphoma cells. Compare the cells in Figures 9 and 10 to adjacent polymorphonuclear leukocytes to assess cell size. Lymphocytes and polymorphonuclear leukocytes make excellent measuring sticks for determining the size of tumor cells, if one remembers that the latter measure about 8–10 μ in diameter.

The nuclei show some pleomorphism, and some of the nuclei have nuclear lobulations. Nearly all of the nuclei show clear areas interrupted by a coarse nuclear mass, which, in some areas, accumulates along the nuclear membrane. The tumor section seen in Figure 1 reveals considerable nuclear pleomorphism. No keratin was found, but intercellular bridges were noted. Compare these cells with Plates 18 and 19, which were described as having keratin and intercellular bridges. Note that the cells from this plate are smaller and basophilic, while the keratinizing cells of Plates 18 and 19 are larger, orangeophilic, and more pleomorphic.

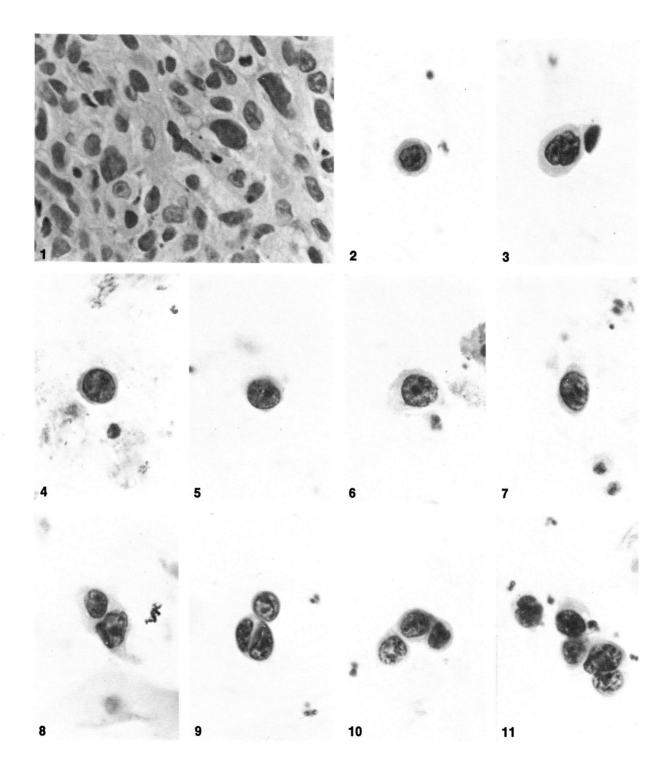

Plate 24

CARCINOMA, SQUAMOUS
(WHO IC)

This 46-year-old patient had smoked cigarettes since the age of 15 and had mined uranium and other hard rock for 20 years. Sputum studies revealed tumor cells (Figs. 3–6), and chest X-rays revealed a mass in the right upper lobe with right hilar involvement. Other sputum samples taken prior to surgery revealed numerous tumor cells (Figs. 7–14). These cells were very subtle and difficult to diagnose because they were rather small (Figs. 6, 8, 9, 11, 14), measuring 15–40 μ, but others were large and degenerate (Figs. 3, 5) with basophilically stained cytoplasm. Some of the cells were elongated (Figs. 3, 5, 10) and, with the basophilic cytoplasm, simulated degenerating abnormal columnar cells. Careful search of all tumor cells, however, revealed two significant features. First, the cells seemingly belong to a family—all have dark nuclei with coarse nuclear substance and basophilic cytoplasm. Second, the cells are very pleomorphic, and many of them show prominent acidophilic nucleoli (Figs. 3, 5, 6, 9, 10, 12, 13). All of these features confirm the diagnosis of malignancy. The histology (Figs. 1, 2) revealed an undifferentiated squamous cell tumor with numerous mitotic figures. The right upper lobe was resected and revealed a tumor mass which measured 3 cm in diameter.

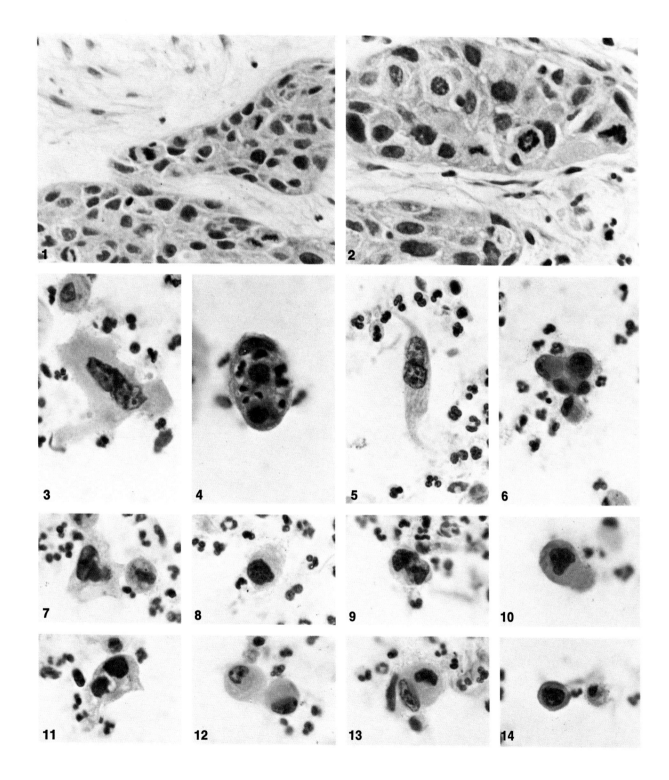

Plate 25

CARCINOMA, SQUAMOUS
(WHO IC)

This tumor developed in the left main stem bronchus of a 76-year-old male who was a very heavy cigarette smoker (4 pkg/day). Histology of the tumor reveals masses of squamous cells with very little fibrous supporting stroma. The cells are held loosely together, and no evidence of keratin or intercellular bridges is found. The cells are small (15–25 μ in diameter), show all shapes, and have prominent irregularly shaped nuclei that vary in size (Fig. 1).

The abundant cells found in sputum from these patients are usually seen in pairs, as in Figures 2–6, with a rather pronounced increase in the nuclear/cytoplasmic ratio and small rim of basophilically stained cytoplasm. The nuclear material is coarse and darkly stained with hematoxylin. Generally, the nuclear membrane is smooth, as seen in Figures 2–5, 7, and 8, but it is angled in Figures 6, 9, and 11. Acidophilic nucleoli are large (Figs. 2–6, 8–11). These nucleoli are also seen in the sections, but are less conspicuous.

It was stressed in Plate 6 that abnormal columnars can sometimes be misleading and interpreted as malignant (false positive) cells. Here we should caution that sometimes these malignant cells may be interpreted as abnormal columnars (false negative). These tumor cells are about the same size or smaller than the unusually large, ballooned, degenerating, abnormal columnar cells, but the smaller degenerating columnar cells are within the same size range as these tumor cells and may create a diagnostic dilemma.

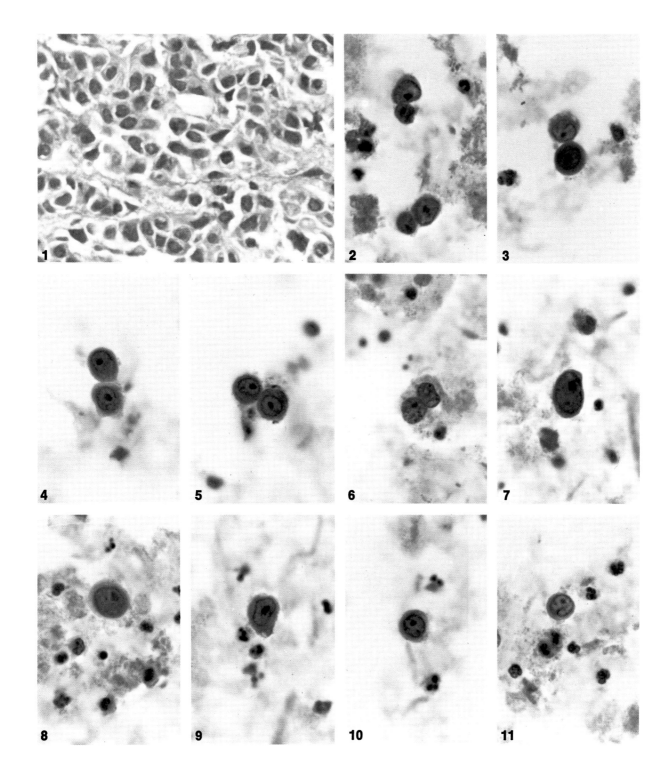

Plate 26

CARCINOMA, ADENOSQUAMOUS (WHO V), AND CARCINOMA, SMALL CELL (WHO IIA)

This is the case of a 56-year-old uranium miner who smoked 1½ packages of cigarettes daily for 30 years. The progression of cytology is shown in Figures 1–8. Figures 1–4 show gradual progression—Figure 2 is a picture taken one year after Figure 1, and Figures 3 and 4 were taken two years later. Figures 5–8 show a variety of cells seen in the last year or five years after the initial changes, and probably all represent malignant cellular elements. This, of course, is most prominent in the huge orangeophilic cell seen in Figure 8 with the classical malignant features of coarse nuclear material, nuclear membrane protrusions, a wrinkled membrane with clefts and accumulated masses of nuclear material, and clear zones in the nuclear matrix.

An adenosquamous cell tumor (WHO V) was found in the upper lobe of the right lung at autopsy. The cells in Figure 11 were found admixed with the epidermoid cells and represent a second anaplastic cell tumor (WHO IIA), seen here in Figure 12. This primary was found in the left lower lobe. The cells photographed in Figure 10, which are larger than those in Figure 11, probably represent the adenosquamous cell component of the tumor seen on the section in Figure 9. Those seen in Figure 11 are small, measuring 10–12 μ in diameter, and were shed by the tumor demonstrated in the section in Figure 12, showing the second small cell tumor.

Although double tumors are rare, nonetheless, we must be alert to this possibility, particularly if repeated specimens are being examined in assessing effectiveness of therapy or in patients that may have been exposed to multiple carcinogens.

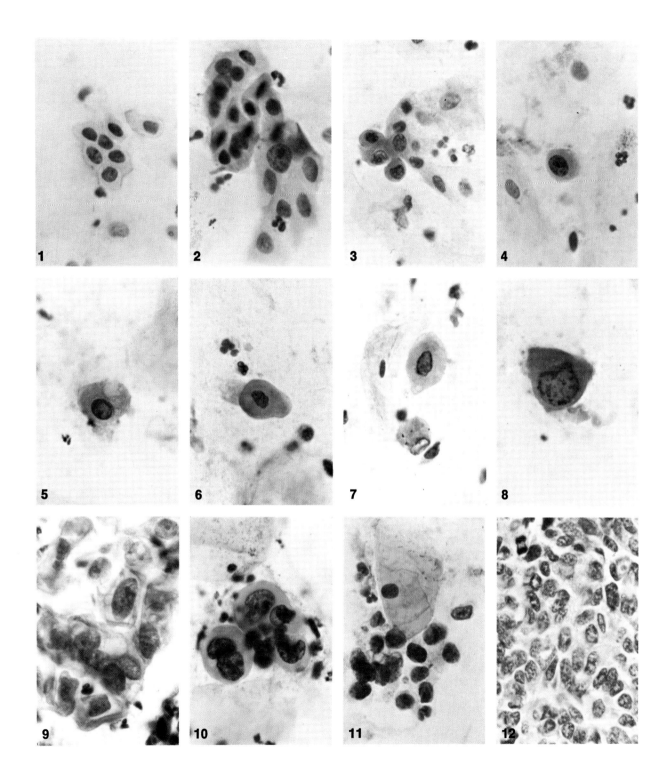

Plate 27

CARCINOMA, SQUAMOUS
(WHO IC)

This 68-year-old male developed a tumor in the left lung, which rapidly extended to involve both lungs with numerous nodules. The tumor, on section (Fig. 1), shows a mixture of squamous cellular elements consisting of nests of squamous cells with no evidence of pearl formation or intercellular bridges. There are also smaller cells intermingled with the others. It is interesting to note that the cells found in the sputum also revealed these two cell types. Figures 2–8 show small (10–15 μ) cells that form clusters or syncytia. The cells have hyperchromatically stained nuclei that also show molding, particularly those in Figures 3, 5, 6 and 7.

The other cells found in the sputum are much larger (20–25 μ in diameter) with abundant, basophilically stained cytoplasm, and the nuclei are coal black. The cell nests show some molding (Figs. 9, 10).

This tumor, like many others that reveal a variety of cells, confirms the thesis that no two tumors, even of the same cellular type, are exactly the same. Each, like its bearer, has its own personality.

68

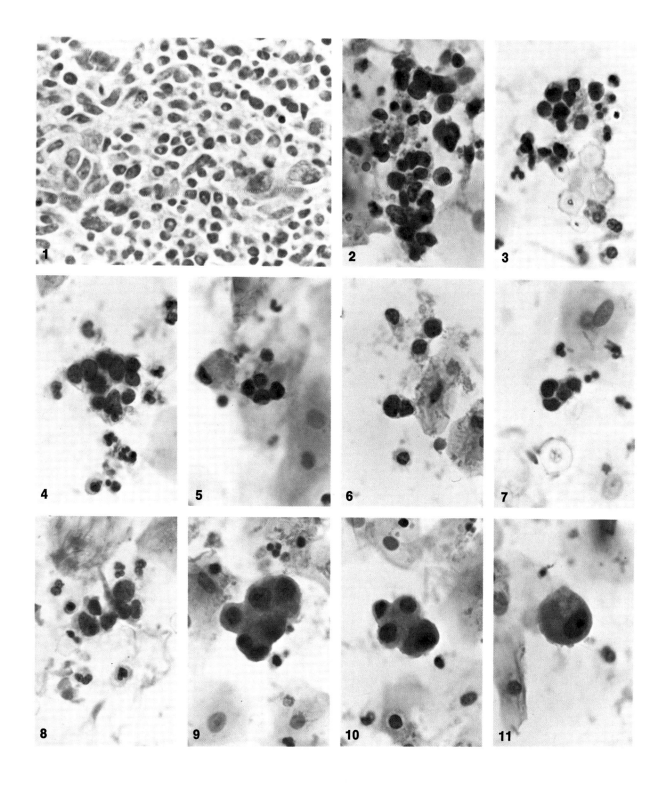

Plate 28

ADENOSQUAMOUS CELL CARCINOMA (WHO V)

This tumor is from the hilar area of the left lung of a 48-year-old real estate salesman who had smoked two packages of cigarettes a day for 25 years. Sections of the tumor in this case reveal a variety of cells, predominantly of squamous cell type (Fig. 1), supported by abundant fibrous stroma. These tumors usually do not produce keratin but do show intercellular bridges. Some areas of the tumor are composed of glandular structures presenting a mixed pattern, which is PAS negative. The cells exfoliated in sputum by these tumors are usually large, measuring 50 to 90 μ or more in diameter. The case presented here has rather basophilic pleomorphic cells with prominent nuclear material. Rare vacuoles (Fig. 2) are noted. The cytoplasm is abundant, and some of the cells show acidophilic nucleoli (Figs. 7–9). Usually these cells are abundant. If they are rare the diagnosis must be guarded because cells, such as noted in Figures 5 and 6, are elongated and simulate abnormal, degenerating, tall columnar cells. The acidophilic nucleoli, however, support the criteria of malignancy.

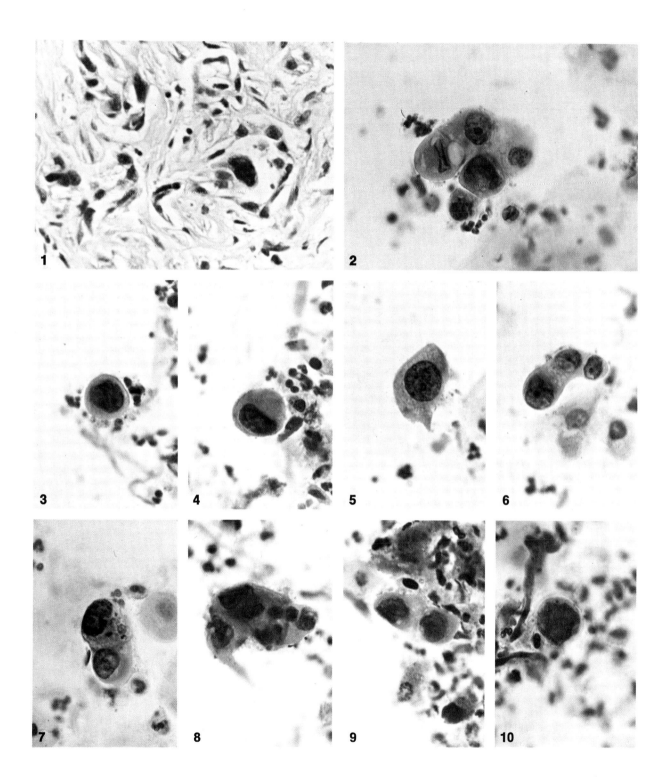

Plate 29

ADENOCARCINOMA, BRONCHOGENIC, PAPILLARY (WHO IIIA-2)

This tumor is from the left upper lobe of a 50-year-old male college teacher who had never smoked. This is an adenocarcinoma (bronchiolar) that originated in a peripheral scar of the left upper lobe (Fig. 4). This type of tumor accounts for 5–9% of the lung tumors in men and 49% in women. Many of these lesions are seen in noncigarette smokers, and many develop in scars. The scars may be of any etiology, but are often the result of a primary Ghon lesion. Adenocarcinoma is very common in Japan and could represent the residuum of healed tubercular lesions. Fibrocytes and fibroblasts are still identifiable in the scar. The tumor was small (2 cm) and barely visible on X-rays. The tumor adjacent to the scar formed prominent, rather large glands lined by cuboidal to transitional-like cells with prominent acidophilic nucleoli (Figs. 1–3).

Metastatic tumor was found in the most peripheral nodes of the lobe (Figs. 5, 6), but the nodes of the mediastinum were without tumor. The cells found in the sputum were usually seen in clusters (Figs. 7, 8, 9). Figures 7 and 8 are the same cluster but photographed to show different planes of cells in focus. Smith and Frable[1] interpret this clustering as diagnostic of tumor since it suggests that this is the tip end of a papillary process. There usually is no molding of cells or nuclei since these processes are not under pressure. Single cells, all with acidophilic nucleoli, were also noted. In addition, rare vacuoles that may represent cellular degeneration (Fig. 11) were seen. Most of the cells range from 30 to 45 μ in diameter, but some are elongated as seen in Figure 12. Although regional lymph node metastases were found, this man shows no recurrent disease after four years.

REFERENCE

1. Smith JH, Frable WJ: Adenocarcinoma of the lung; cytological correlation with histologic types. Acta Cytol 18:316–320, 1974.

72

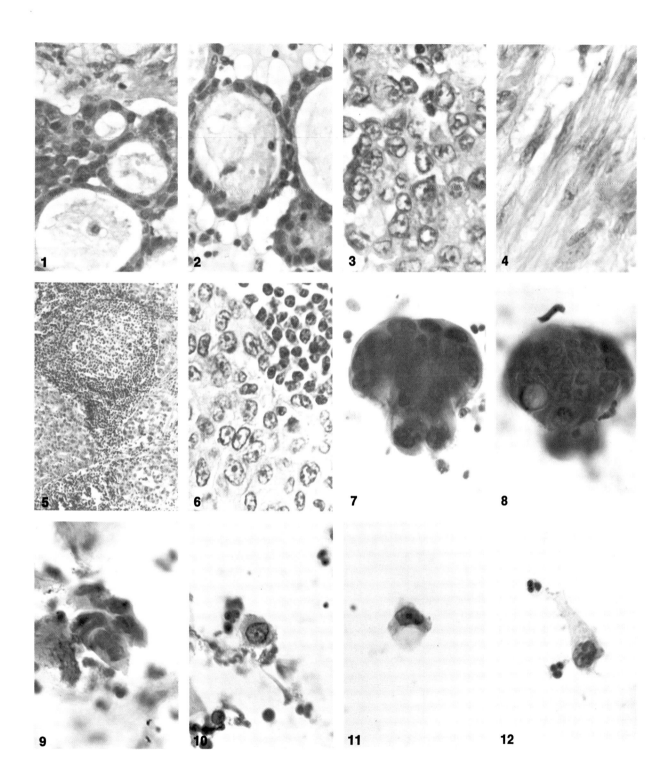

Plate 30

ADENOCARCINOMA, BRONCHOGENIC, PAPILLARY (WHO IIIA-2)

This tumor developed in the left lower lobe of a 62-year-old male who mined uranium for many years and was a heavy cigarette smoker. These tumors, like all true adenocarcinomas, account for 5 to 9% of all lung neoplasms in males and again are frequently found in scars or, on occasion, in peripheral lung parenchyma. The histology of these tumors varies considerably, depending on the position of origin. If the tumors arise in the true small bronchioles, they are classically adenomatous, showing characteristic glandular structures. On the other hand, if these tumors arise more peripherally in the smaller bronchioles or alveolar spaces, the glandular structures may not be abundant, and the dilated respiratory areas seem to blend with alveolar spaces. The tumor tends to migrate along respiratory-lined septa, which simulate respiratory areas. The true alveolar tumors, if such an entity really exists, show little or no bronchiolar arrangement.

These tumors, as is noted in Figures 1 and 2, show bronchioles lined by tall columnar cells that in some areas appear to crowd the epithelium to form a papillary process projecting into the lumen. Secretory vacuoles are seen frequently in the sections, especially in the lining cells but are rarely seen in exfoliated cells except for vacuoles of degeneration, as is seen in Figures 3 and 5. Most of the exfoliated cells are seen in clusters and obviously are fragments of the lining papillary protrusions. The cells are molded, usually measure 15 to 30 μ in diameter, and almost always show acidophilic nucleoli.

74

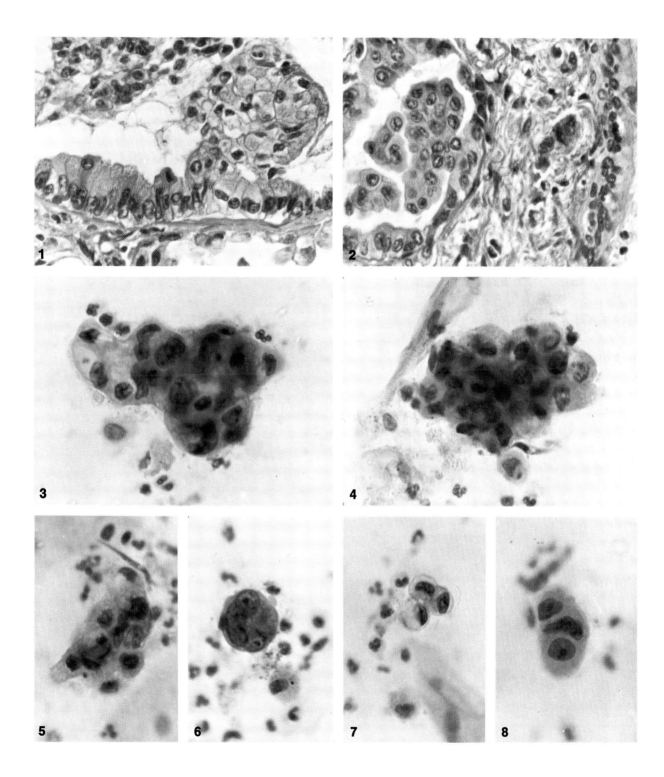

Plate 31

ADENOCARCINOMA, BRONCHIOLO-ALVEOLAR (WHO IIIB)

This lung neoplasm, found in the left lower lobe of an 83-year-old male, shows a varied histology, demonstrating a mixed bronchiolo-alveolar pattern. These tumors may have a preponderance of either bronchiolar, papillary, or alveolar cells, depending on the type of pattern that dominates the histology. Cytologically, this tumor shows alveolar adenocarcinomatous cells.

Figure 1 shows papillary processes supported by a fibrous core that modifies the lining cells into glands and protruding processes covered by tall columnar goblet cells. The primary solid area is small and extends to involve the surrounding respiratory bronchioles but especially the alveolar spaces. The tumor not only lines these spaces but forms protruding processes which project into these alveolar spaces, as shown in the section seen in Figure 2. The cells in Figures 3–6 are clustered into sheets, which are processes that have become free of their attachment along the alveoli and still cling together. Occasional free cells are found (Fig. 3), and these show secretory vacuoles or vacuoles of degeneration. The vacuoles are noted in many of the cells. As noted in Figure 6, some of the cell nests show marked cellular degeneration with extensive nuclear and cytoplasmic fragmentation. Many of the nuclei show all of the nuclear malignant features, primarily hyperchromatism and pleomorphism.

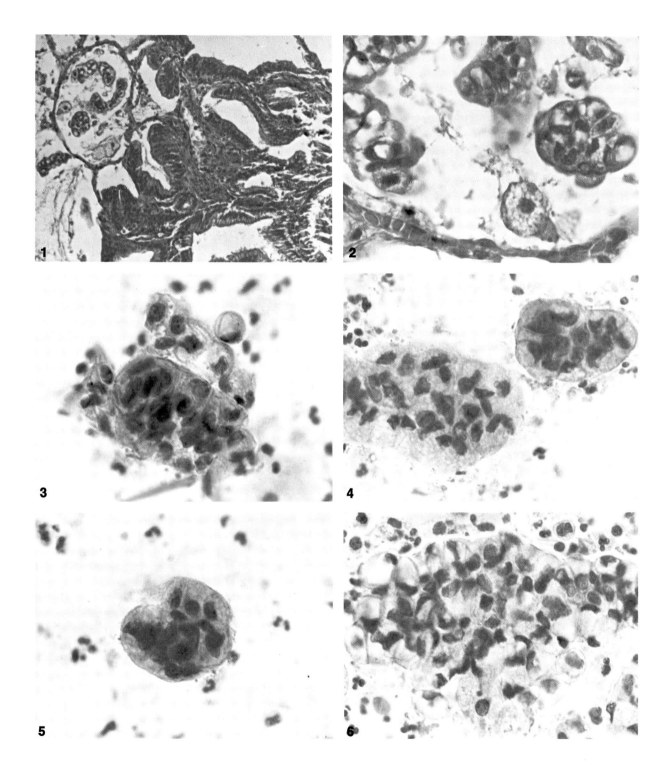

Plate 32

ADENOCARCINOMA, BRONCHOGENIC (WHO IIIA-1)

This tumor developed in the right middle lobe of the lung in a 60-year-old male patient who smoked three to four packages of cigarettes per day for 40 years. Adenocarcinomas account for 5–9% of the lung neoplasms in males and nearly half of the malignant lesions in females. They usually arise in the peripheral portions of the lung and frequently develop in peripheral scars. Some of these tumors, however, are true adenocarcinomas developing in glands in the submucosa. The tumor in this case is of this latter type and probably should be defined as a true gland tumor (WHO VII), but these are difficult to separate from the WHO IIIA types. These lesions protrude into the bronchial tree and shed cells into the bronchial stream. The tumors are PAS positive and are composed of numerous glands lined by tall columnar cells, which show basally placed, rather regular nuclei and a very clear cytoplasm. The supporting stroma is composed of very loose areolar connective tissue.

Cells found in the sputum vary considerably in size, measuring 15 to 60 μ in diameter, and the nuclei are usually deeply stained and stand out on the usual orangeophilic sputum smear. The cytoplasm is basophilically stained, and this also adds to the dark, conspicuous character of these cells. The cells may be found in clusters (Figs. 3–8) or may be single (Fig. 11). Usually, they are single. Figure 2 shows phagocytosis. The cytoplasm, as seen here, is bluish, abundant and usually not vacuolated, although vacuoles are seen (Fig. 6). The nuclei are round but may show angulation, and the nuclear material is finely granular with uniform distribution. Prominent, rounded, eosinophilic nucleoli are seen in many of the cells.

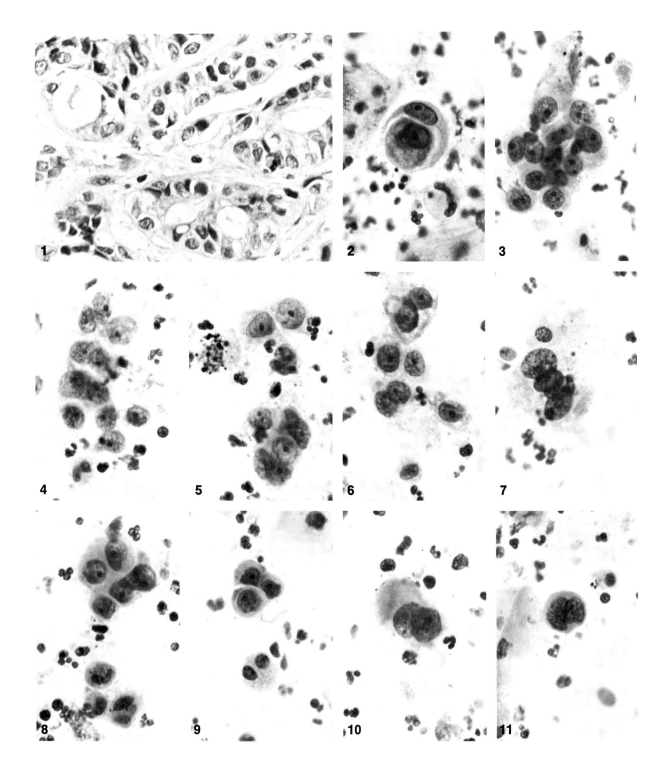

Plate 33

ADENOCARCINOMA, BRONCHOGENIC (WHO IIIA-1)

This case of cancer of the lung is interesting because it presents one of the shortcomings of sputum cytology as an adjunct in establishing a definitive diagnosis of cancer in peripheral scar lesions. Fortunately, not all of these lesions are so obstinately reluctant to shed cells in the sputum.

This 52-year-old female had smoked two packages of cigarettes a day for 30 years. She had a chronic cough of several years duration accompanied by hoarseness. Approximately three years prior to the definitive diagnosis of malignancy, three specimens revealed a marked atypical squamous cell metaplasia. Finally, an ill-defined lesion in the left upper lobe was identified on X-ray, and it remained essentially the same for about two months, but the sputum continued to be negative. Eventually, a portion of the left upper lobe was removed, and sections revealed a classical scar adenocarcinoma (Fig. 1). A year later, sputum samples taken on several occasions were positive (Figs. 3–12), and the X-rays at this time revealed a bilateral lung nodularity. Finally, central nervous system pathology resulted in a craniotomy in the left temporal area, involving removal of a nodule that was metastatic adenocarcinoma (Fig. 2).

When the sputum cytology became positive, it was seen that all of the cells had a basophilic cytoplasm, were large, being 30–50 μ in diameter, with some even larger and elongate (Fig. 3). The nuclei were lobulated, deeply stained and some revealed acidophilic nucleoli (Figs. 4–7).

Initially, the sputum cytology did not yield a positive diagnosis in this case, and it is cases like this that have given sputum cytology in peripheral lesions a very poor diagnostic reputation. Although we have not made a statistical study of the positive cases in our peripheral lesions, we have been impressed that most cases of this type will yield a positive diagnosis even early in the development of these tumors, particularly the bronchiolar and alveolar types. This tumor may have developed from submucous glands and may not have communicated with the bronchiolo-alveolar areas, which is always necessary if shed tumor cells are to be found in the sputum.

80

Plate 34

ADENOCARCINOMA, BRONCHOGENIC, PAPILLARY (WHO IIIA-2)

This tumor was removed from a 65-year-old female who was a non-cigarette smoker with a chronic productive cough. This is another variant of peripheral respiratory adenocarcinoma—the bronchogenic papillary type. Sputum studies revealed an abundance of single and clustered exfoliated cells, many of which showed vacuoles of degeneration, although the cells appeared to be very well preserved (Figs. 3, 4, 8). These cells vary markedly in size from 15 to 80 μ in diameter and show molding, but the molding is not striking in most clusters. Some cells reveal acidophilic nucleoli as the tumor spreads peripherally from the central core, which is sometimes very firm and may be an old scar. The cells seem to spread along the alveolar lining and form papillary fronds that project into these spaces, eventually completely filling the alveoli. This process gradually replaces respiratory areas, reducing respiratory reserves.

At surgery, no mediastinal metastasis or regional lymph node involvement was found, and a left lower lobectomy was done. The lesion was primarily peripheral, but nearly all of the lobe revealed small to large foci of tumor extending along respiratory and alveolar walls. Histologically, it was a mixed bronchogenic adenocarcinoma of papillary cell type (WHO IIIA-2). No other metastatic lesions have been discovered, but three years after surgery, the patient had positive sputum and obvious bilateral disease revealed by X-ray, with recurrent cough and shortness of breath.

This is another example of tumor developing in a scar in a non-cigarette smoker. Histologically, these tumors vary only slightly, but no two appear exactly the same. The manner in which these tumors spread, whether or not metastasis is found, varies markedly in small or large tumors. As a result, the prognosis is varied and therefore unpredictable. In this case, there was a rather extensive involvement of the excised lobe but no regional or distant metastases, and the tumor spread was slow and localized. In other cases with slightly different histology and cytology tumors have spread rapidly by lymphatic and blood metastases. See Plate 33 for a case involving brain metastasis.

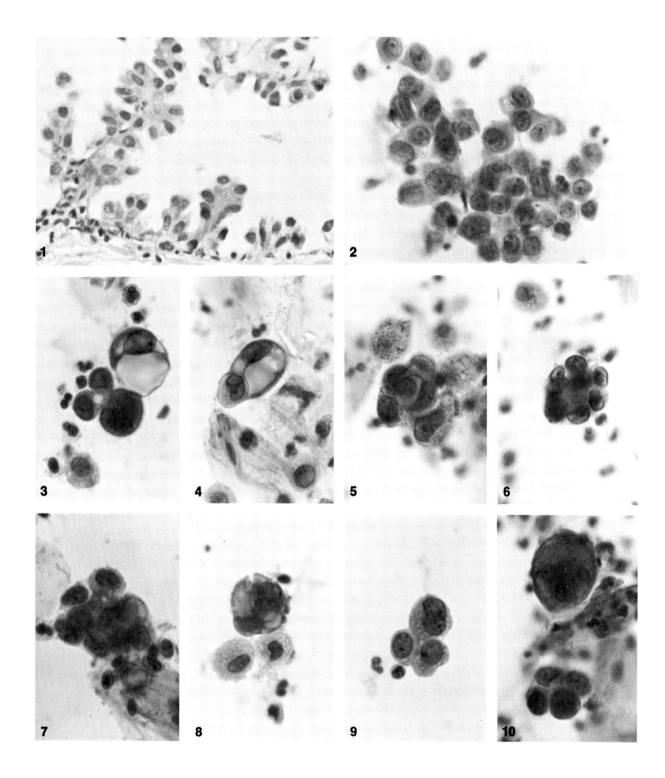

Plate 35

LARGE CELL (GIANT), UNDIFFERENTIATED CARCINOMA OF THE LUNG (WHO IVB)

This tumor is from the lung of a 74-year-old male patient who had smoked 30 cigarettes daily for 57 years. The tumor is from the right upper lobe. Interestingly, the patient's primary complaints were referable to his gastrointestinal tract and included a 15-pound weight loss. On admission, routine X-rays revealed the tumor, and sputum cytology revealed abundant tumor cells. The sections of the tumor showed cellular characteristics typical of this lesion, and the nuclei exhibited changes more pronounced than usual. Note the two large nuclei in the large cells. The nuclear membrane shows indentations, breaks, mouse bites, and the nuclear material accumulates along the membrane in clusters. In addition, the nuclear matrix is coarse and breaks an almost clear nuclear background. The nucleoli, particularly in the smaller nucleus of Figure 1, are large and have a roughened surface. Even the nuclei of the smaller cells seen in Figure 2 exhibit these malignant features. All of the cells in these tumors characteristically vary in size, shape, and nuclear matrix. Moreover, they seem to be floating in an invisible matrix with very little supporting stroma.

The cells found in the sputum samples are numerous and show features similar to those seen in the tumor. Some are very large, measuring over 100 μ in diameter (Figs. 3, 10, 11), while others are very small (Figs. 4–7). The cells all stain basophilically with dark nuclei, only a few of which reveal the nuclear substance. This bizarre pattern is characteristic of these tumor cells.

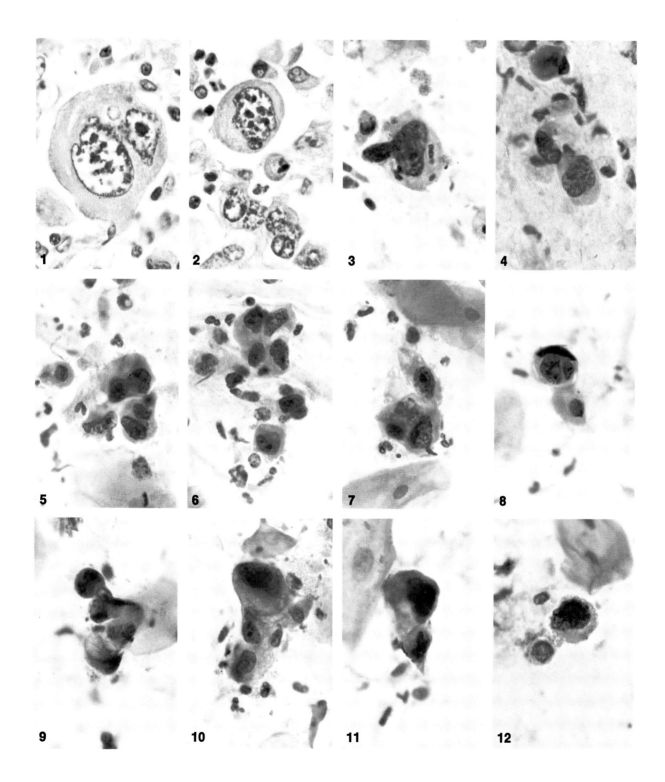

Plate 36

LARGE CELL (GIANT), UNDIFFERENTIATED CARCINOMA OF THE LUNG (WHO IVB)

This large cell, undifferentiated carcinoma is from a 67-year-old construction foreman with a history of smoking three packages of cigarettes per day for many years. This type of lesion accounts for about 5% of lung neoplasias, and these tumors are usually peripheral in position. They are unique histologically because of the variation in cell size. Most of the sections of these lesions show a squamoid appearance with primarily undifferentiated, relatively small cells which simulate WHO IC or B, but this pattern is interrupted by large cells as noted in Figures 1 and 2. The cells on section appear loosely arranged and sometimes appear to be nonadhesive and floating in a fluid matrix. A similar cellular pattern is seen in the sputum samples. Some large cells are noted (Figs. 3, 5, 6, 7), with some of them reaching dimensions of over 200 μ in diameter, while other cells are rather regular in size and shape, may be paired, but are small (15–20 μ). Many of the cells appear to be giant cells with multiple nuclei (Figs. 3, 8, 9). One wonders if the small cells are not previously a large giant cell which had separated into an aggregate, as noted in Figure 4, while Figure 3 shows a huge single cell with abundant cytoplasm. Some of the cells are positive for mucin. Cell phagocytosis is frequently seen in this lesion.

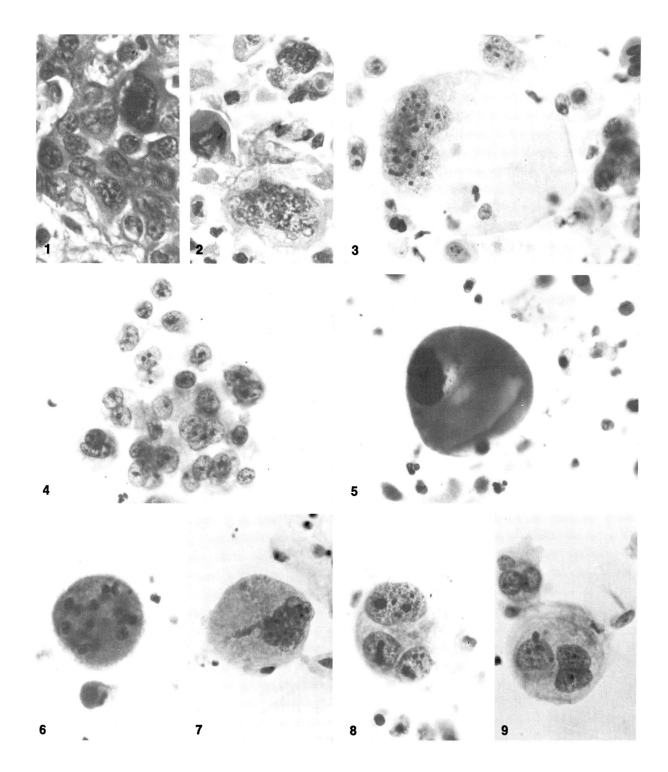

Plate 37

COMBINED CARCINOMA

ADENOCARCINOMA, PAPILLARY (WHO IIIA-2) AND SQUAMOUS CARCINOMA (WHO IB)

This mixed or double (squamous and adenocarcinoma) tumor of the lung is seen in 0.5% of all malignant lung lesions. This lesion, measuring 3.5 cm in diameter, was in the right lower lobe and arose in the main stem bronchus. It was not recognized by sputum cytology as having a double cell pattern of adenocarcinoma and squamous cell type. The tumor was mixed adenosquamous in the midzone, but as the periphery was approached, it was composed entirely of squamous tumor cells. The other half of the tumor revealed an entirely glandular pattern. The two histological patterns are seen in Figures 1 and 2, respectively. The cytological patterns observed in the sputum revealed numerous dark single cells (Figs. 3, 4, 6–9, 11–16), but occasional paired cells were noted. The glandular cell elements were rather large, 25–40 μ in diameter, and most of the cells revealed ill-defined, degenerating cytoplasm. Some of the cells appeared elongated and basophilic, suggesting a glandular pattern. No vacuolation is seen in the cytoplasm, and the nuclei are composed of coarse nuclear fragments with prominent nucleoli (Figs. 3–8, 11, 12, and 16). Figures 17 and 18 reveal orangeophilic cells which may be from the squamous portion of the tumor. These cells were not numerous and poorly preserved, unfortunately making it difficult to identify them as malignant. Some of these tumor cells, as seen in Figures 7, 10, 11, 12, and 15, are quite elongated and may be erroneously mistaken as abnormal columnars, but this is excluded by their nuclear structure.

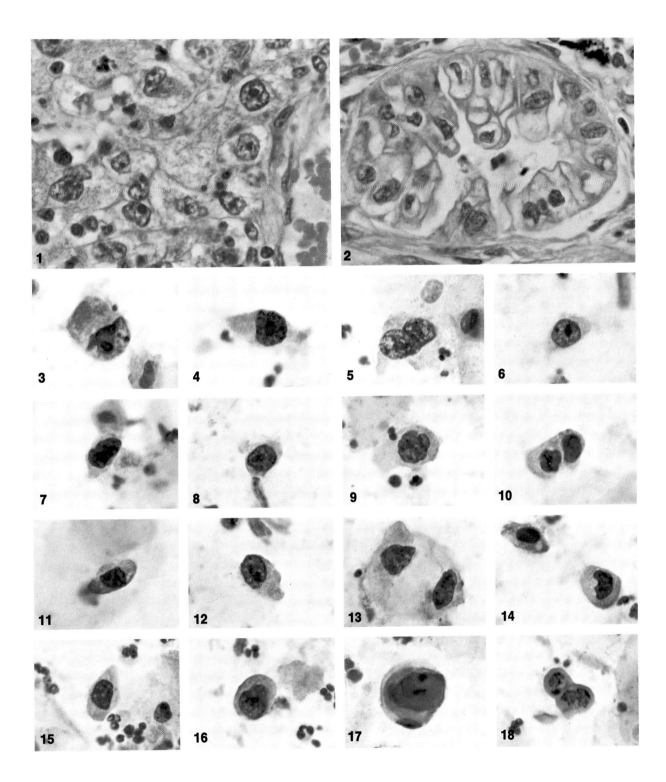

Plate 38

CARCINOMA – DOUBLE TUMOR

SQUAMOUS (WHO IA) AND SMALL CELL (WHO IIA)

This is a double tumor from a 63-year-old cigarette smoker (2 pkg/day/50 years), who had been a coal miner for 9½ years. He developed shortness of breath, and chest X-rays revealed a large right hilar mass with fluid in the right costophrenic angle. Sputum cytology revealed the variety of cells shown here (Figs. 2–16), and aspiration of the pleural effusion yielded the cells seen in Figures 17–19.

Examination of the sputum reveals a variety of cells (Figs. 2–16). Those in Figure 2 are small, measuring 10–15 μ in diameter, and the nuclear material is coarse. All of the cells are of about the same morphology but bound into tight clusters, except for the cells seen in Figures 13, 14, 15 and the large cell in Figure 17. These cells are larger – 20 μ in Figures 13 and 14. The cell in Figure 15 is a huge keratinizing cell, which measures more than 50 μ in length. These cells are orangeophilic, show nucleoli and coarse nuclear material and therefore suggest epidermoid carcinoma. The large cell seen in Figure 17 supports this diagnosis. All of the other cells, including those from the pleural fluid (Figs. 17–19), show small cell tumor.

Fiberoptic bronchoscopy revealed a tumor in the right main stem bronchus, and biopsy showed both tumors – an epidermoid (WHO IA or B) and a small cell tumor (the dark cells, WHO II, Fig. 1). It is unusual to see two cytologically different tumors in a patient at the same time but even more unusual to see both tumors in a 2-mm biopsy taken by fiberoptic bronchoscopy.

90

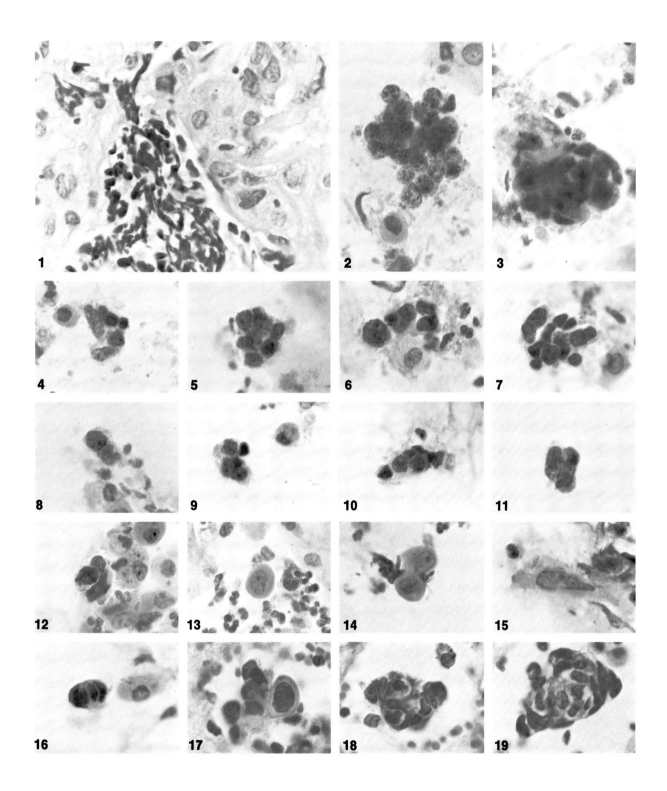

Plate 39

CARCINOMA—DOUBLE TUMOR

SQUAMOUS (WHO IA) AND SMALL CELL (WHO IIA)

This is a very interesting case with an unusual tumor combination found in a uranium miner who died at age 56. He was a heavy cigarette smoker. Sputum cytology at age 53 revealed the variety of epidermoid tumor cells seen in Figures 4–9. The cells were large and keratinized (Figs. 5–8), and the nuclei were characteristically malignant. X-rays did not show tumor at this time. Fiberoptic bronchoscopy was not available at that time, but rigid bronchoscopy failed to reveal a lesion. He was hospitalized again at age 55 for urinary infection and reevaluation of his diabetes. A chest X-ray was taken at that time and revealed a linear infiltrate in the left mid-lung field. A month later, he was readmitted for bronchoscopy and sputum studies. Physical examination revealed a Virchow's node on the left and a few palpable lymph nodes in the right supraclavicular area. The sputum revealed numerous nests of small cells (Figs. 10–11) which measure 10–20 μ in diameter with hyperchromatic nuclei and very little cytoplasm. These were identified as small cell carcinoma (WHO IIB).

At autopsy and serial block section study, the left lower lobe revealed the two tumors seen in Figure 1. The section in the left field reveals epidermoid carcinoma (WHO IA), while the right portion shows small cell carcinoma. Figure 2 is a higher power view. Figure 3 reveals a carcinoma in situ showing two unusually large nuclei. This was located in the left upper lobe.

Two cell types, both invasive, are not usually seen in one tumor. Usually the tumor of one cell type will appear in one lung, while the other may be in the opposite lung or even in a different lobe of the same lung. These tumors will be growing at different rates and will usually vary in size. Lukeman (personal communication) noted a small portion of a little (less than 1 cm in diameter) oat cell tumor, which revealed a small islet of epidermoid carcinoma near one margin. Since the oat cells grow so rapidly, one would assume that the epidermoid lesion, growing at a much slower rate, would be lost in the final histology of the tumor. The keratinizing cells, seen in sputum long before small cells develop, suggest that multiple carcinogens may be eliciting different types of cellular changes, or possibly the same carcinogen may cause a reaction on different target cells producing two varied responses.[1]

REFERENCE

1. Saccomanno G: Atypical metaplasia of the bronchial epithelium; frequency and significance, a preliminary report. (Unpublished)

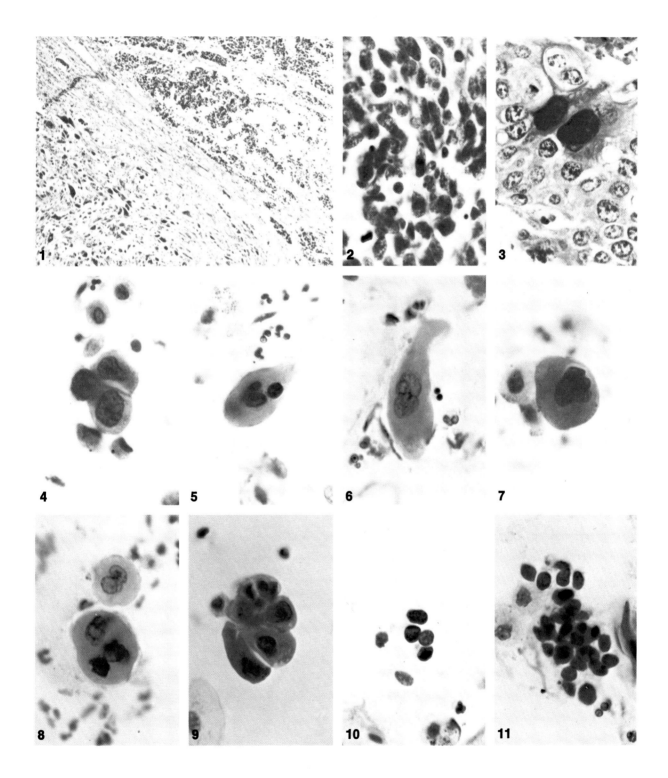

Plate 40

LYMPHOCYTES

Lymphocytes are rare in noninflammatory sputum samples and common in sputum from patients with pulmonary viral infections. They are, however, sometimes seen in abundance in primary or metastatic lymphomas involving the lung. Observation of abundant lymphocytes in sputum should always alert one to check for systemic lymphoma. The cells may be single, in clusters, or streamers, as seen in all of these figures. Some of the lymphocytes are bilobed and are thought to be an effect of radiation. See Figure 8, which was from a uranium miner who was exposed to radon daughter radiation.[1] The lymphocytes that show nuclear detail, such as those seen in Figure 6, reveal a fine vesicular to fine granular pattern and are readily identified as typical and benign, but do vary slightly in size. Some of the nuclei, however, are coal-black and slightly pleomorphic, as seen in Figures 4, 5, 7, and 8. These are suspicious and may be confused with small cell (oat cell) carcinoma, which has cells of similar size. Continued search usually shows cells in which nuclear material can be evaluated, and a correct differentiation will result.

REFERENCE

1. Ingram M: The occurrence and significance of binucleate lymphocytes in peripheral blood after small radiation exposures. Int J Radiat Biol (special supplement) June, 1959

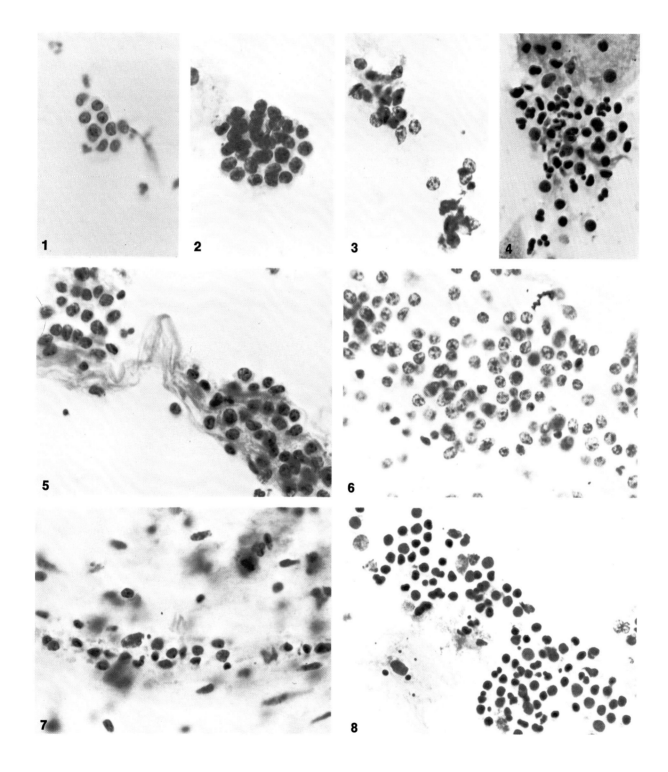

Plate 41

SMALL CELL (OAT CELL) CARCINOMA (WHO IIA)

This tumor developed in the left lower lobe of a 53-year-old miner who had smoked two packages of cigarettes per day for many years. These small cell lesions of the lung have been divided into two and sometimes three varieties by the World Health Organization. When many sections are made of these tumors, invariably all three cell types are found, and the clinical behavior, prognosis, and response to therapy are the same in all three types. It seems then that these lesions should be appropriately grouped into "small cell" type.

Small cell carcinoma is a lesion frequently seen in very heavy cigarette smokers and accounts for about 19% of the malignant lesions of the lung in non-miners who smoke cigarettes. The incidence in uranium miners is higher (35%). It is thought that cigarette smoking causes squamous cell metaplasia, which is then vulnerable to the radiation carcinogen, initiating the tumor. This hypothesis, however, may be questioned for two reasons. First, it has been suggested by many writers that small cell carcinoma is of neurogenic cell (Kulchitsky) origin.[1] Second, we have reviewed the tracheobronchial trees of many patients who died from small cell carcinoma, and we have been unable to show any cells suggesting that small cell tumors do indeed originate from the epithelial lining, either normal or metaplastic. Nonetheless, the carcinogenic effect of radiation cannot be denied in the presence of such a high incidence of disease in the uranium miner. In any event, these tumors are clinically the most aggressive of all the neoplasms of the lung, elicit no immune response, sometimes secrete a variety of hormones, and run a very rapid course. Treatment of small cell tumors with chemicals and radiation shows some promise, however.

The histology is usually uniform (Fig. 1), but at times some squamous-like areas are found. The sputum smears vary considerably and are usually not too difficult to diagnose. Usually, the cells are in clusters or streamers, as shown in Figures 2–14. The cells are small, varying from 8–20 μ, and frequently the nuclei are coal black (Figs. 4, 5). However, search among these cell nests will reveal well-preserved nuclei that have classical coarse nuclear substance with wrinkling of the nuclear membrane. Notching and bilobulations are also noted (Figs. 5, 6). Another feature, which is frequently seen in these lesions and should always arouse suspicion, is nuclear debris, indicating cell fragmentation (Figs. 4, 5, 6). In diagnosing these lesions, the most common error is calling lymphocytes small tumor cells, rather than failing to identify small cell tumors.

REFERENCE

1. Hattori S, et al: Oat cell carcinoma of the lung — Clinical and morphological studies in relation to its histogenesis. Cancer 30:1014–1024, 1972

96

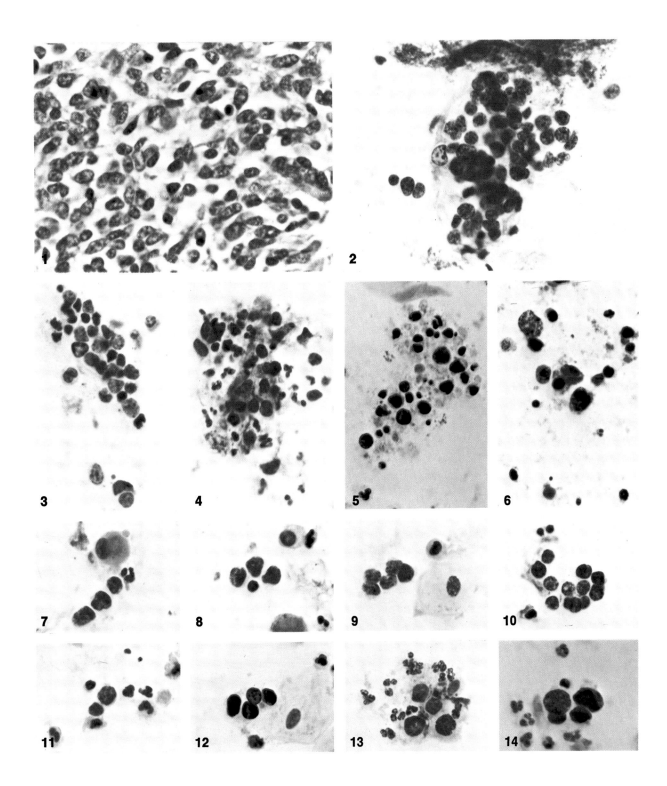

Plate 42

SMALL CELL CARCINOMA OF THE LUNG (WHO IIB)

This case involves another small cell tumor of the lung showing slightly more pleomorphism histologically. This patient, a uranium miner, smoked cigarettes for 40 years. The cells in this lesion are slightly larger and, in some areas, appear to show a squamoid pattern and form sheets which closely resemble undifferentiated squamous cell carcinoma of the WHO IC variety. This shows well-preserved cells with no evidence of necrosis, at least in the area photographed here. Necrosis is frequently seen in these small cell tumors, and would therefore be expected in the positive sputum samples. Small fragments of cells are seen in Figures 3, 5, and 6. This material is called nuclear debris. The cells seen in Figures 2–6 are either free cells or sheets of cells, and close inspection of nests of these cells reveals a fine mesh of mucin binding them to each other. The tumor cells show very little cytoplasm, and the most prominent feature identifying them as tumor is the nuclear pleomorphism. Occasional cells will show sufficient coarse nuclear material to also be an identifying aid. This is also true of malignant lymphoma cells found in sputum, but the odd shapes and coarse borders identify the cells in this case as of small cell type of lung origin.

This tumor in this case should be classed as an oat cell carcinoma (WHO IIB). Frequently, it is difficult to classify these lesions as either IIA or IIB, because both types of cells, oat cell and polygonal cell, are seen in the same tumor. A similar difficulty is encountered in the cytology of these tumors. All small cell tumors of the lung respond in the same way to radiation and chemotherapy; therefore, one suspects that these tumors are essentially the same, and it is suggested that they be categorized as one tumor (WHO II).

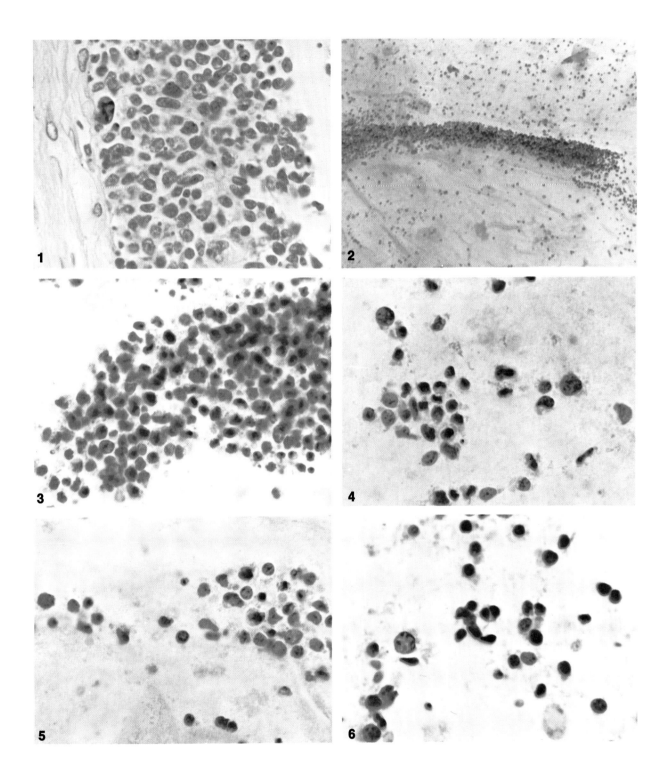

Plate 43

CARCINOID (WHO VI)

This 50-year-old female patient had had two episodes of hematemesis but otherwise had been well. Sputum studies were not done, but bronchial washings revealed benign small cells described below. The tumor was visible on X-ray as a solitary lesion in the left lower lobe bronchus, and sections of the excised tumor revealed a typical benign pattern seen in Figures 1 and 2. Much speculation about the origin of these tumors has been presented recently, and there still is some question as to the cell of origin. Most of the evidence is that these lesions are argyrophilic, but not argentaffin.[1] Bronchial carcinoid syndrome is characterized by severe and prolonged flushing, apparently because carcinoids produce histamine and 5-OH tryptophane instead of serotonin.[2]

Since these tumors often protrude into the bronchi, it is surprising that cells are not shed from the surface and found in sputum samples. The bronchial wash sample (Figs. 3–10) reveals single cells and clusters of cells, varying in size from 12–18 μ in diameter. The nuclei vary slightly in size and shape, are basophilically stained, and the nuclear substance varies from fine vesicular to coarse granules, but all of the nuclei appear the same otherwise. The nuclear membrane is smooth and no nuclear accumulations are noted, which is also consistent with a benign cellular pattern.

The primary lesion was removed, and no recurrence has been noted in five years.

REFERENCES

1. Anderson WAD: Pathology, ed 6. St. Louis: CV Mosby Co, 1971, p 980
2. Frank HD, Lieberthal MM: Carcinoid syndrome originating in bronchial adenoma. Arch Int Med 111:791–798, 1963

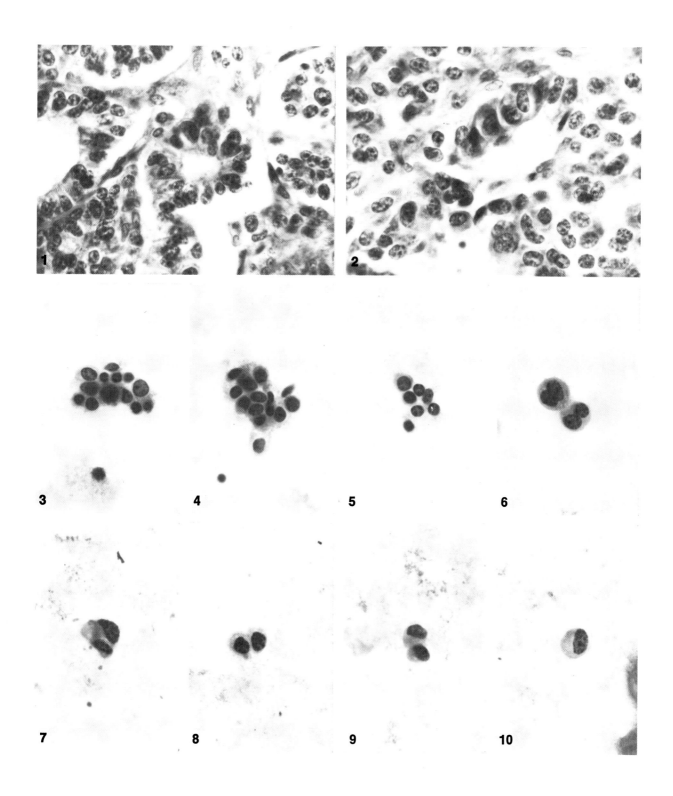

Plate 44

LYMPHOMA, HISTIOCYTIC (RETICULUM CELL SARCOMA), PRIMARY LUNG (WHO VIIIC)

Scattered mononuclear cells are seen frequently in sputum samples and probably represent a normal element of the cellular component of these samples. When these cells are found in increased numbers, it must be determined if they are normal, active lymphocytes that are seen in the viral pneumonic process or if the cells are of a malignant variety. Numerous studies must be made to confirm the diagnosis of lymphoma. Physical findings, chest X-rays, bone marrow studies, or even lymph node biopsy should be done to confirm systemic disease. Primary lymphomas of the lung may remain as localized lesions for many years or involve the mediastinum and grow very slowly.

The case presented here was observed clinically for a 14-year period. On X-ray, a lesion in the right middle lobe was first noted at age 59, but the patient refused treatment. Fourteen years after the initial diagnosis of lung tumor, he developed a chronic cough, had a 20-pound weight loss, and the right lung lesion was enlarged with obvious mediastinal involvement. At this time, sputum samples revealed numerous small cells (Figs. 2–10). The cells were in clusters or syncytia, varied in size, and some showed coarse nuclear substance with some pleomorphism and occasional mitotic figures. Most of the cells simulated lymphocytic blast cells. A biopsy (Fig. 1) revealed a histiocytic malignant lymphoma. It is difficult to diagnose the specific type of lymphoma from sputum cells, and it should always be confirmed by biopsy to establish the absolutely correct diagnosis for the administration of the most effective chemical or radiation therapy.

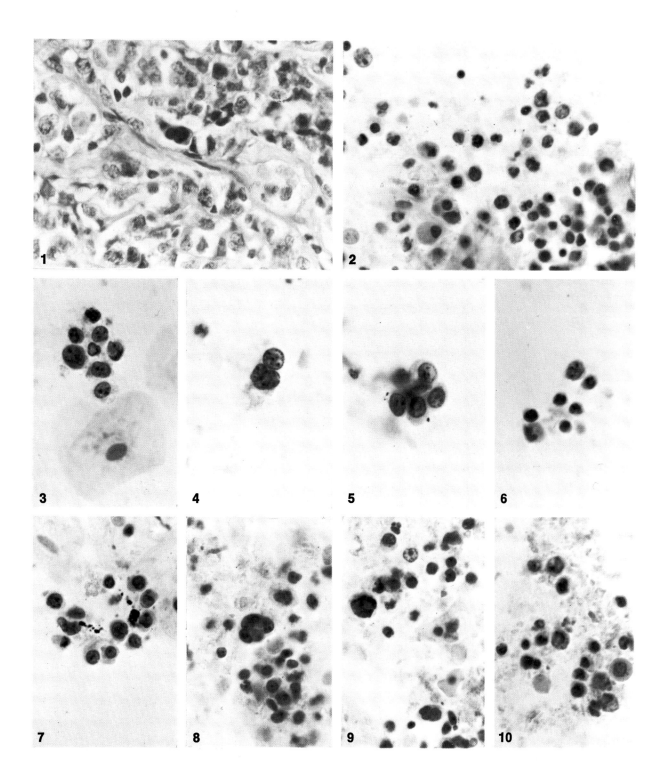

Plate 45

MESOTHELIOMA, RIGHT PLEURA, MALIGNANT (WHO VIIID)

Mesotheliomas are lesions that involve the lining of the major body cavities. Asbestos workers show an increased incidence of both cancer of the lung and mesotheliomas.[1] Slightly more than 50% of mesotheliomas are malignant, and the most common variety is the fibrous type. Tumor cells were found in the pleural fluid in two of the following three cases, which are presented here for that reason. Other articles reveal more detailed histological data.[2]

Two lesions representing different varieties of mesothelioma are shown here. The first is a malignant mixed variant and the second, a malignant fibrous type. Another lesion, also malignant but of the diffuse variety, is shown in Plate 46. The patient in this latter case had tumor cells in the sputum following surgery. Patients with these tumors rarely, if ever, show tumor cells in the sputum prior to surgery, but frequently these cells will appear in the pleural fluid as shown in the first case of this plate and in the case presented in Plate 46. No cells were demonstrated in the second case presented here.

The fibrous benign types usually have thickened fibrous areas and usually do not shed cells into the body cavities. Unfortunately, little can be done in these cases after a diagnosis of neoplasia is made.

The first case was of a 64-year-old patient hospitalized for treatment of intestinal bleeding. A routine admission chest X-ray revealed a wide band of pleural thickening in the right chest with a small amount of fluid in the right costophrenic angle, posteriorly. A small amount of fluid was aspirated and smears revealed the variety of cells seen in Figures 3–9. The cells varied in size from 25 to 40 μ and stained deeply with hematoxylin. The nuclei were basophilic and revealed only a small amount of particulate material, which presented diagnostic problems. Some of the cells were vacuolated (Fig. 8) while others were arranged in clusters. One nest (Fig. 9) suggested a glandular pattern. A biopsy was taken which revealed a mixture of various features (Figs. 1, 2). Some areas were tubular as seen in Figure 1, while others were more cellular. The cells in both areas were pleomorphic and revealed numerous mitoses. Exposure of this patient to asbestos was not ascertained.

The second case was of a 63-year-old male patient who developed a thickened band, visible with X-ray, in the right lung field. Exploration of the chest in this area revealed a thick firm meaty band of tumorous tissue over the lung with nodules over the pericardial visceral pleura. Histologically, the tumor (Figs. 10 and 11) revealed spindle cells with some pleomorphism. Prominent acidophilic nucleoli are noted in many of the cells. The lesion is a fibrous variety with low grade malignancy. This patient had a three-year exposure to asbestos as a miner.

REFERENCES

1. Hourihane DO: The pathology of mesotheliomata and an analysis of their association with asbestos exposure. Thorax 19:263–278, 1964
2. Stout AP, Lattes R: Atlas of Tumor Pathology, Second Series, Fascicle I, Tumors of the Soft Tissues—Malignant Mesotheliomas. Washington D.C.: AFIP, 1966, pp 176–178
3. Kauffman SL, Stout AP: Mesothelioma in children. Cancer 17:539–544, 1964
4. Winslow DJ, Taylor HB: Malignant peritoneal mesotheliomas: a clinicopathological analysis of 12 fatal cases. Cancer 13:127–136, 1960

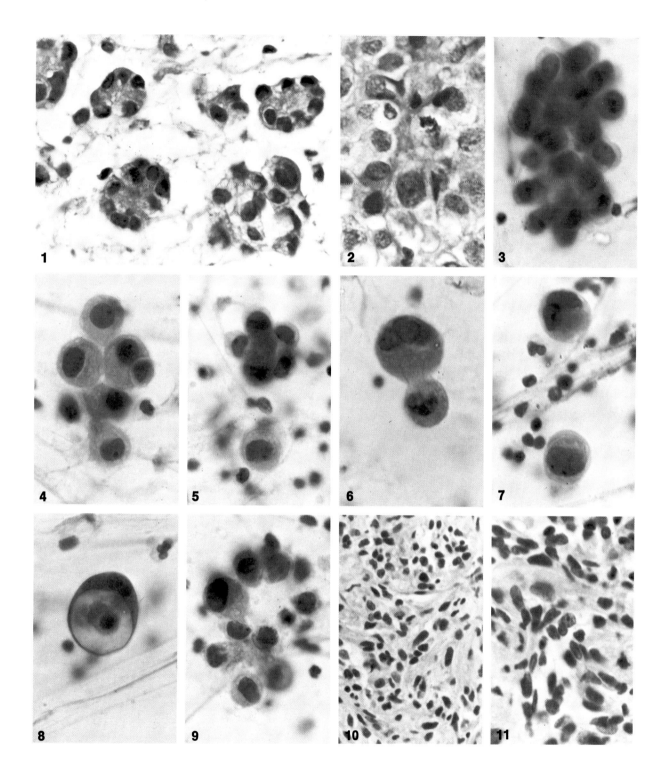

Plate 46

MESOTHELIOMA (WHO VIIID)

This 53-year-old patient developed chest pain. He had never been an asbestos worker. On X-ray, a lesion was found in the right chest. Pleural fluid was present, and examination revealed the cells seen in Figures 6, 7, and 8. Subsequent to biopsy of the lesion (Figs. 1, 2), tumor cells were found in the sputum (Figs. 3, 4, 5). These cells were seen singly and in clusters and measured $30-40\,\mu$ in diameter. All showed a marked increase in nuclear/cytoplasmic ratio and showed some cytoplasmic degeneration. The patient was treated with chemicals and radiation, which resulted in some clinical improvement, but he eventually developed pleural effusion and died of cardiac complications.

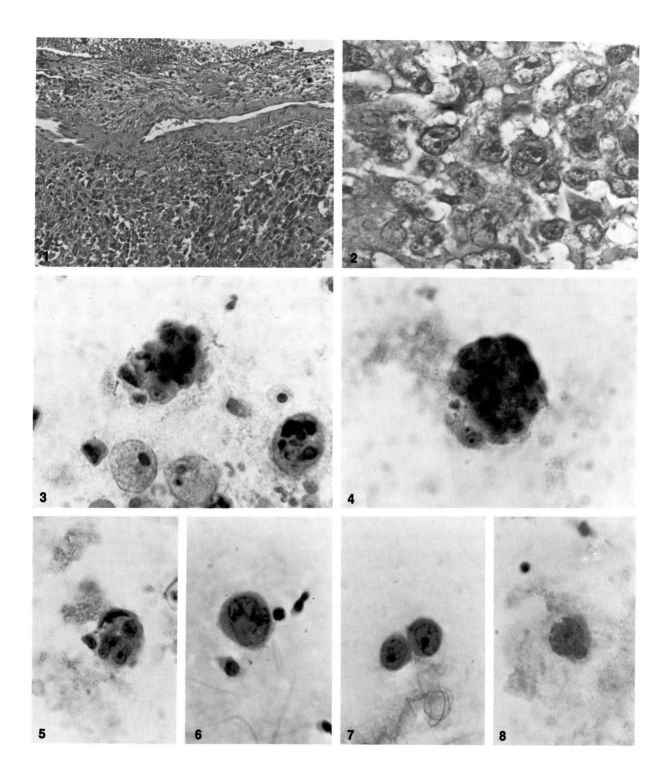

Plate 47

LYMPHOMA, LYMPHOCYTIC, DIFFUSE, METASTATIC OR EXTENSION FROM MEDIASTINUM

Primary lymphosarcoma of the lung is a rare disease. Metastatic lymphosarcoma involving the lung is a late complication of generalized disease, and cells from lung involvement may be found in the sputum of patients with disseminated disease.

Figure 1 is a section of an enlarged lymph node from a left upper mediastinal mass, visible on X-ray, from a 41-year-old male. The sections were identified as lymphosarcoma, diffuse lymphocytic type. Sputum studies revealed the variety of lymphocytic cells and abundant tumor cell debris seen particularly in Figures 3 and 4 and in smaller amounts in Figures 2 and 5. The lymphocytic cells vary in size in the smears as they do in the section of the node. Some of the cells are large, measuring 15 to 18 μ in diameter (Fig. 5) with adjacent cells measuring less than 8 μ in diameter. The nuclear material is coarse, and this appears to be more prominent in the larger nuclei. The cytoplasm is scanty and hardly detectable in these photographs. The diagnosis of lymphosarcoma with lung involvement was confirmed with the presence of these cells in the sputum. The patient was treated with radiation therapy and survived five years.

It may often be difficult to distinguish these cells from those of other small cell tumors. Acidophilic nucleoli will aid in distinguishing oat cells from malignant lymphocytic cells, and cells of lymphoid origin, although pleomorphic, usually have round nuclei. The reader should compare these cells.

108

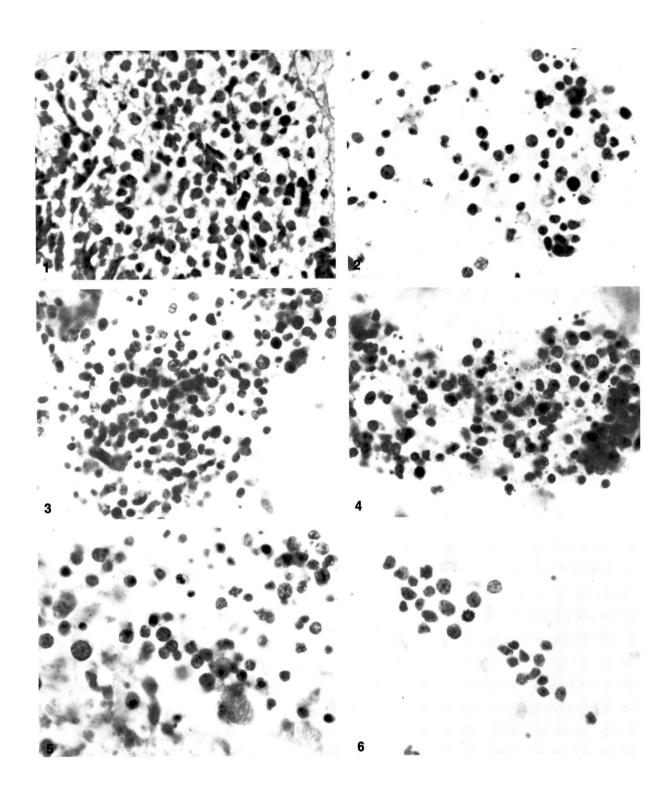

Plate 48

CARCINOMA, SQUAMOUS, CERVIX, METASTATIC TO LUNG

This patient, a 47-year-old nurse, had a positive cervical Pap smear for squamous cell carcinoma. Cervical conization confirmed the diagnosis of invasive squamous cell carcinoma that was large cell and nonkeratinizing. The patient was treated with radium implants but a year later showed recurrence of the tumor on the posterior vaginal wall. X-rays of the chest, following a positive diagnosis of malignancy from sputum studies, revealed bilateral lung metastases. Figure 1 is a section of the positive cone. Figures 2 and 3 are positive imprint smears made from the lung metastasis, and Figures 4–10 are cells found in sputum samples prior to death. The tumor cells found in the sputum show some shrinkage and loss of detail of the nuclear material. However, they are still identifiable as malignant, although it may be difficult to identify the primary tumor from these cells. Patients who have had malignant disease and show clinical signs of its recurrence, such as loss of appetite, weight loss, or fever of long duration, should have a sputum cytological examination. Sometimes, the earliest signs of disseminated tumor are confirmed by sputum cytology. Moreover, if the sputum cytology is positive, it justifies aggressive chemotherapy. A positive sputum cytology may confirm recurrence in patients considered to have minimal residual carcinoma.

110

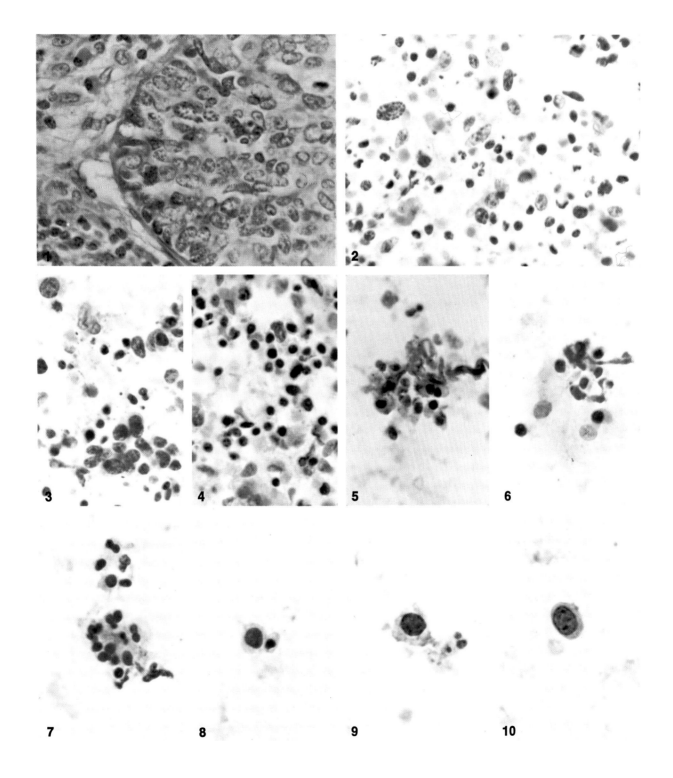

Plate 49

ADENOCARCINOMA, BREAST, METASTATIC TO LUNG

Breast cancer, common in females, is a lesion with many varieties having different clinical responses to surgery, hormone therapy, and chemotherapy.[1, 2] Early diagnosis, of course, improves the prognosis; but once a diagnosis of carcinoma of the breast is established, the clinical course of the disease is very unpredictable. One hopes that the surgery has removed all of the tumor and that the patient is cured, but no method of establishing that the disease has been unequivocally removed is available. In reality, 60–80% of these patients do not have recurrent disease, but the remaining 20–40% do eventually have recurrences, and the latter are considered to have "minimal residual disease." Recurrence will occur at various sites—locally at the site of the original excision or distally in the axilla, bone, liver, ovary, lung, etc. Frequently, in lung involvement lesions are visible on X-ray but not always, and in either event, confirmation of the recurrence may sometimes be made with sputum cytology. Positive sputum cytology, of course, indicates a serious state of advanced disease and justifies aggressive chemotherapy. Once this therapy has been administered, the sputum will become negative if the treatment has been effective. Frequent sputum cytological examination can be an effective adjunct to identification of clinical symptoms in the monitoring of breast tumor recurrence.

The cases presented here represent three varieties of breast tumor. The histological sections are on the left, and the six figures on the right show the positive cytology found in the sputum of these patients with recurrent disease.

The first case (Fig. 1) involves the histology of a breast tumor (duct cell carcinoma) from a 69-year-old patient who had the tumor removed at age 66. She was well for three years, but then bilateral lung nodularities were revealed. Sputum studies showed the variety of cells in Figures 2–7. The cells are rather large, measuring 30–50 μ in diameter. They may be single but are usually seen in tight clusters. Some nuclear molding is present (Fig. 5), and the cells are basophilically stained with dark nuclei. Some of the cells show prominent acidophilic nuclei (Figs. 3, 4, 6). The cells in duct adenocarcinoma are larger than those in lobular or medullary adenocarcinoma.

Figure 8 is a section of lobular adenocarcinoma from a 53-year-old patient who showed axillary metastasis at surgery. Sputum cytology was positive two years after the primary surgery, and X-rays at this time were also positive. The tumor cells in this patient's sputum are small, measuring 20–30 μ in diameter, forming tight clusters with nuclear molding (Figs. 9, 12, 13). Again, like the cells seen from other breast tumors, these are basophilically stained, both in the nucleus and cytoplasm. Figure 10 reveals signet-ring cells, which Steinbrecher[3] reported as a characteristic often seen in breast tumor but more frequently in the lobular type of carcinoma. These cells are sometimes difficult to identify because the clusters are small and may be missed on screening.

Figure 15 is a section from a right breast tumor of a 43-year-old woman. The carcinoma remained quiescent with minimal residual disease for 22 years. The only apparent recurrence was pulmonary. The primary lesion was medullary adenocarcinoma. X-ray revealed recurrence bilaterally in the lungs. The sputum was positive (Figs. 16–21), showing numerous clusters of tightly bound tumor cells that again showed basophilic staining with nuclear molding.

REFERENCES

1. McDivitt RW, Stewart FW, Berg JW: Tumors of the Breast, in Atlas of Tumor Pathology, Fascicle 2. Washington, DC:AFIP, 1967
2. Ackerman LV, Rosai J: Surgical Pathology, ed 5. St. Louis: Mosby, 1974, pp 912–930
3. Steinbrecher JS, Silverburg SG: Signet-ring cell carcinoma of the breast. Cancer 37: 828–840, 1976

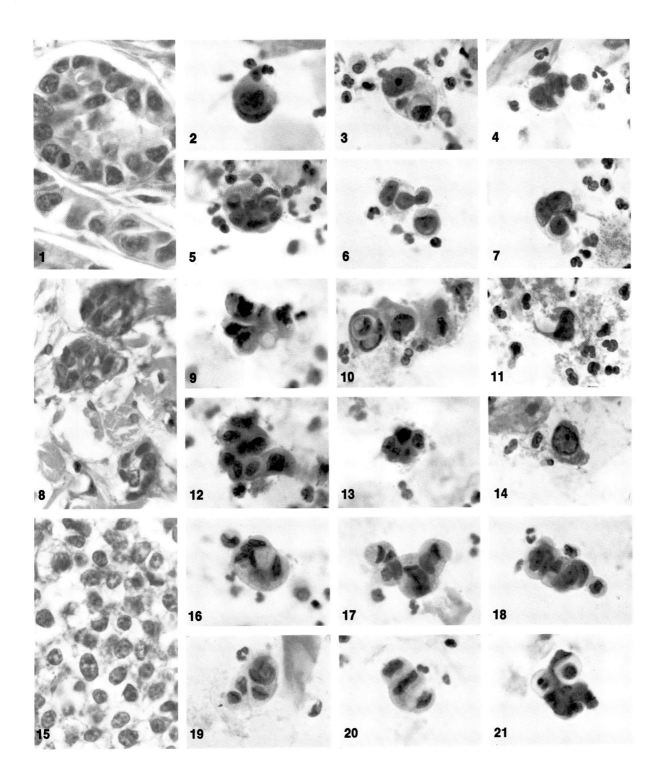

Plate 50

ADENOCARCINOMA, BREAST (DUCT CELL TYPE), METASTATIC TO LUNG

This case of breast tumor is presented because the tumor cells found in the sputum sample reveal a variety of cell types. This lesion was removed from the left breast of a 74-year-old patient who also had a concomitant, similar lesion in the right breast.

Histologically, this tumor is a very cellular duct cell carcinoma (Fig. 1) revealing ducts lined by a variety of cuboidal cells that are very pleomorphic. Even in the photograph, one can observe marked pleomorphism in the huge, deeply stained nuclei and, when compared to some of the smaller nuclei, the cell-size variation is quite extreme.

All of the cells found in the sputum samples from this patient are at the same magnification. Some (Figs. 5, 6, 7, 10, 11) are very large, measuring $50-60$ μ in diameter, while those seen in Figures 3, 4, 14, 21 are very small, measuring from $15-30$ μ in size. All of the cells are basophilically stained, and some show irregularly shaped nuclei with acidophilic nucleoli (Figs. 14, 16). This tumor reveals features similar to the duct carcinoma described on Plate 49, but the cells seen in the sections are more pleomorphic, as noted above.

114

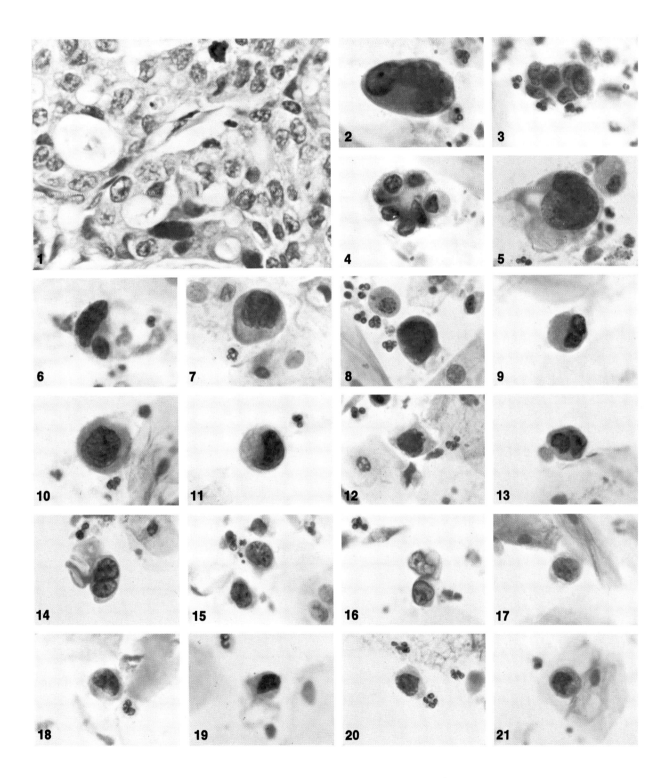

Plate 51

ADENOCARCINOMA, BREAST (MEDULLARY TYPE), METASTATIC TO LUNG

Figure 1 shows a low power micrograph of a section of the primary lesion in the left breast of a 58-year-old patient who was a nonsmoker. Figure 2 is a high power view showing several mitotic cells with very little supporting connective tissue stroma. The remaining figures show cells found in the sputum. Tumor cells are frequently found in sputum of patients showing generalized carcinomatosis, with or without X-ray visible lung metastases. The cells from metastatic tumor of the breast, as seen in Figures 3–10, are well preserved and seen singly or in clusters. They are usually found in clusters in lung involvement and are generally small, measuring 15–25 μ in diameter.

When patients with advanced disease are under chemotherapy, the first indication of response is a decrease or total disappearance of cells in the sputum. Likewise, when therapy is stopped because of clinical improvement, one of the first types of evidence of generalized recurrence is the presence or reappearance of tumor cells in the sputum. Thus, sputum study for tumor cells may be an excellent method of monitoring the effectiveness of chemotherapy.

116

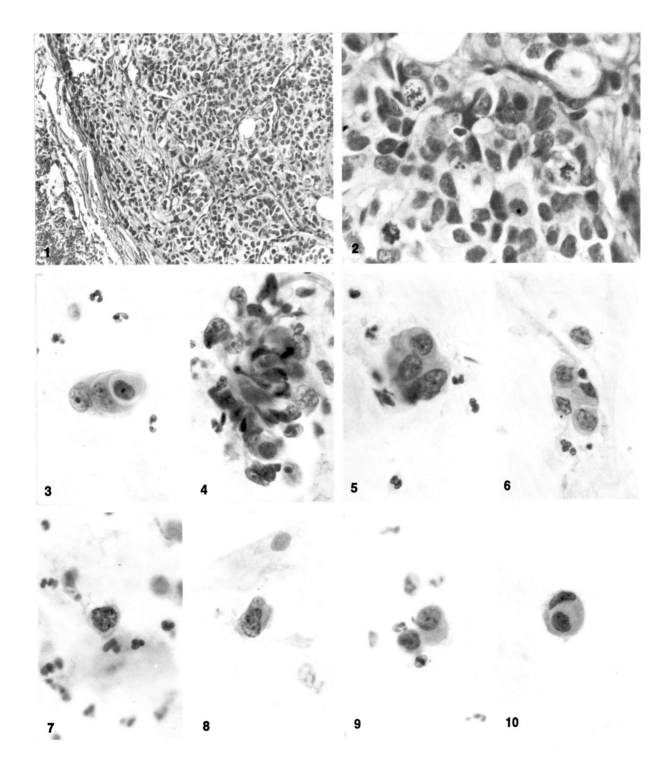

Plate 52

ADENOCARCINOMA, PANCREAS, METASTATIC TO LUNG

This is the case of a 65-year-old male patient with pulmonary metastases from adenocarcinoma of the pancreas. Like other malignant cell metastases, these indicate advanced disease.

Figure 1 is a section of the adenocarcinoma of the pancreas. The sputum cells (Figs. 2–11) exfoliated by these metastatic lesions are usually well preserved and of similar size, measuring approximately 50–80 μ in diameter. The cytoplasm may be scanty and bluish in color, and the cell membrane may show some fragmentation. The nuclear material is rather coarsely granular, and the nuclear membrane is distorted by nubbins, folds, and mouse bites. Some of the cells have prominent acidophilic nucleoli, which often have a roughened surface and are lobulated (Figs. 4, 6, 7, 8, 9, 10). Note the clear areas in the nuclei of the cells in Figures 2, 3, 6, 7, 8, and 11. Usually, these cells, like most metastatic cells to the lung, are easily identified in sputum samples because of their hyperchromatically stained nuclei, regular cell size, and bluish cytoplasm.

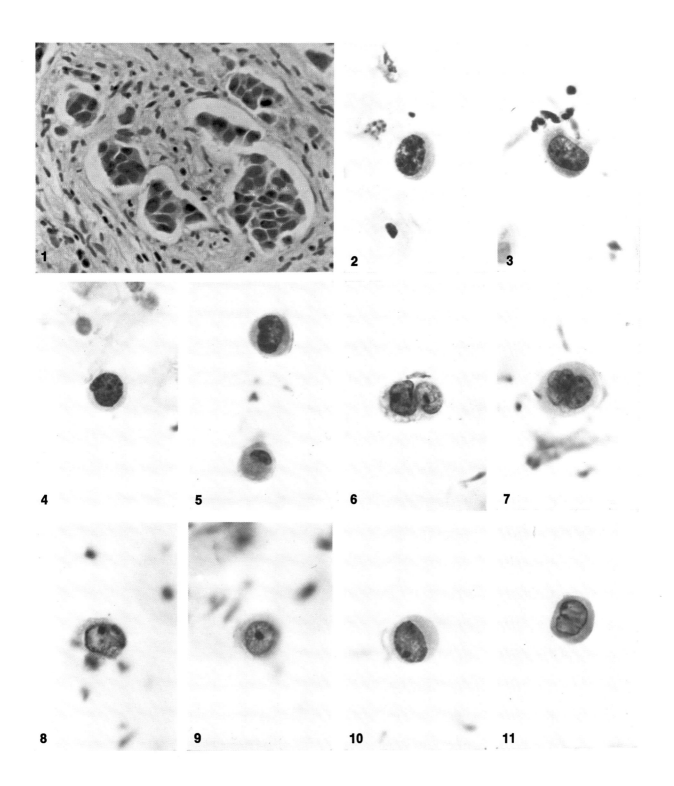

Plate 53

ADENOCARCINOMA, PROSTATE, METASTATIC TO LUNG

This patient was a 67-year-old man who had been a very heavy cigarette smoker for 50 years. Adenocarcinoma of the prostate usually remains localized; however, metastases most frequently occur in bone, but when the disease becomes advanced, spread to the lung may eventually occur, and tumor cells may be found in the sputum.

Figures 1 (low power) and 2 (high power) show photographs of the primary tumor of the prostate. The exfoliated cells seen in the sputum vary in degree of degeneration. These cells and those which are better preserved measure about 20–30 μ in diameter. Some of the cells (Fig. 3) show abundant ghost residual cytoplasm without nuclei. This degenerative process is also noted in Figures 4 and 5, although some of the cells still retain the nuclei which show considerable degeneration with poorly defined nuclear substance. The nuclei vary in size and shape. This is even more pronounced in Figure 6, where the cells are closely adherent. Figures 7–11, however, show the same cells, but the nuclei retain the granular nuclear substance and have the nuclear membrane distortion, allowing one to conclusively identify the cells as malignant. When one observes the ghost anucleated cells, one should suspect tumor and make an added effort to identify these cells by examining more specimens.

A positive sputum smear in this disease usually forecasts a grave prognosis and may indicate aggressive treatment if it has not already been initiated.

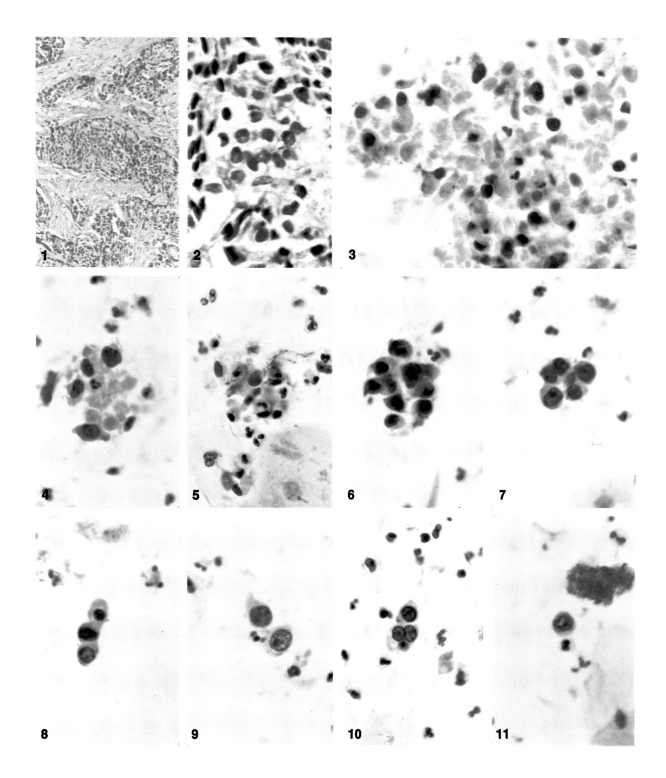

Plate 54

CARCINOMA, TRANSITIONAL, PAPILLARY, KIDNEY, METASTATIC TO LUNG

This neoplasm is histologically similar to the papillary transitional cell carcinoma of the urinary bladder where it is more frequently found. We have not seen this tumor in situ in the kidney, as is sometimes the case in the bladder. Usually, the tumor will mold its architecture within its environment, spreading from the most common site into the pelvis and adjacent calices. Sometimes it may project into the orifice of the ureter and cause partial obstruction in its early stages or even total obstruction, resulting in some degree of hydronephrosis.

Figure 1 (low power) shows the fronds or papillary arrangement of the tumor lined by rather regular transitional cells. Figure 2 (higher power) shows considerable pleomorphism with huge nuclei and coarse nuclear substance, and prominent acidophilic nucleoli. Cells are shed by the fronds into the calices and ureters and may be found in the urine (Figs. 3–5). Again, like lesions in the bladder, these tumors metastasize to the lung. If this occurs, cells are found in the sputum (Fig. 6).

The cells measure about 25–50 μ in diameter and are found in clusters, as shown in Figure 4, or as single cells (Fig. 6). Most of the cells have an increased nuclear/cytoplasmic ratio, and acidophilic nucleoli are seen in a coarse granular nuclear material. Like the metastatic tumor cells from bladder lesions, the nuclei found in the sputum are hyperchromatically stained and are readily identified in sputum samples.

122

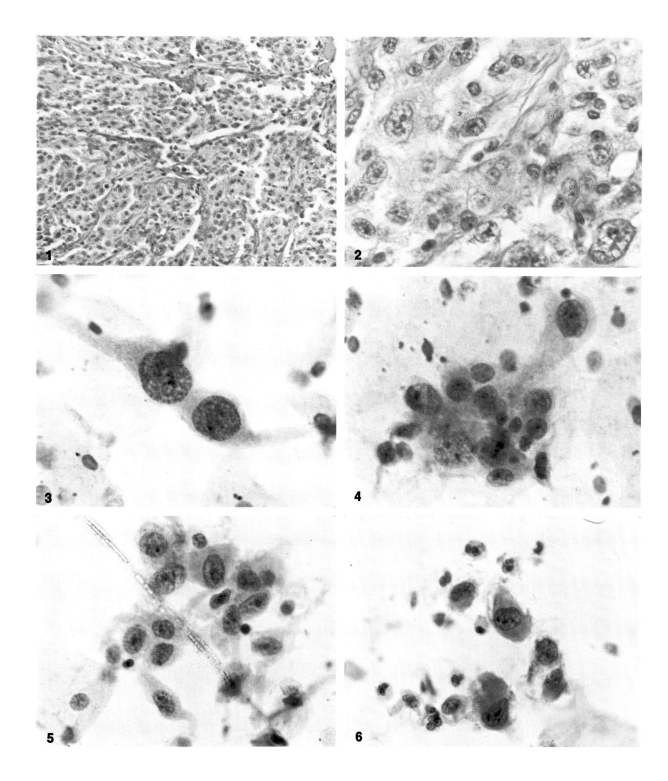

Plate 55

CARCINOMA, TRANSITIONAL PAPILLARY, URINARY BLADDER, METASTATIC TO LUNG

Figures 1 and 2 show a low power and high power view, respectively, of this transitional cell carcinoma of the urinary bladder from a 70-year-old patient. Generally, these tumors are single, although multiple at times, and composed of papillary processes covered by transitional cells of varying degrees of malignancy. Some tumors show soft fronds that are composed of regular transitional cells, while other tumors reveal some regular epithelium admixed with large hyperchromatically stained cells. An occasional tumor will be composed of very anaplastic cells forming solid tumor masses. Transitional cell carcinomas are sometimes in situ lesions. These are difficult to diagnose because the urinary bladder lining appears normal even though the tumor is extensive and shows foci of invasion. Metastases may occur before a lesion is readily recognized in the bladder. Tumor cells from all malignant lesions of the bladder are found in the urine. The more benign tumors yield rather regular cells, making it difficult to differentiate them from normal epithelial cells found in the urine.

These tumors metastasize to the lungs, and these metastases shed cells that are found in sputum. Usually, the tumors that spread to the lungs are of the more aggressive, pleomorphic types and these, of course, shed cells which are of similar morphology, as is shown in Figures 3–10. These cells are usually seen in clusters but are sometimes single, and they measure about $25-50\mu$ in diameter. The nuclear/cytoplasmic ratio is markedly increased, and the cytoplasm has a faint bluish hue. The nuclei are usually deeply stained with nearly complete loss of nuclear detail, although where visible (Figs. 6, 7, 10), the nuclear material is coarse and deeply basophilic. Note the nuclear pleomorphism in Figure 3. The nuclei in Figures 4 and 5, however, are arranged in series, with nuclear molding, and are of uniform size.

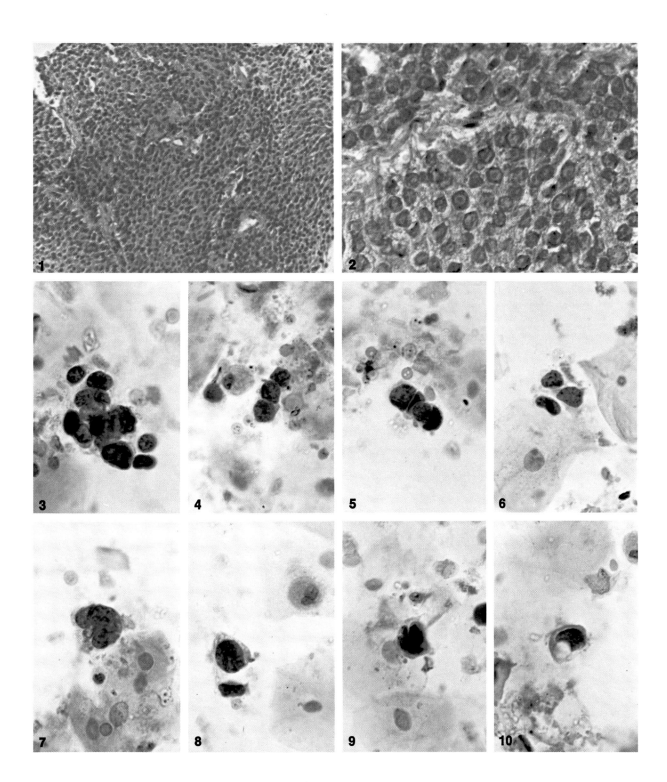

Plate 56

CARCINOMA, RENAL TUBULAR (HYPERNEPHROMA), METASTATIC TO LUNG

This 55-year-old male patient developed a large left kidney tumor and on surgical excision was found to have renal vein invasion. Two years later, he developed a cough, which produced abundant sputum that was positive for metastatic tumor. Chest X-rays also revealed metastatic tumor masses in the upper and lower lobes of the left lung.

The histology of the tumor reveals a classical clear cell hypernephroma (Figs. 1, 2). The cells are arranged in tubular-like structures composed of elongated cells with clear, abundant cytoplasm. The nuclei are rather regular, although some are twice as large as others and show prominent eosinophilic nucleoli. Irregularly shaped nuclei are found, and some have coarse nuclear material.

The tumor cells found in these sputum samples are frequently seen in clusters (Figs. 8, 9, 12), and most of them show more basophilia of the cytoplasm. However, some cells (Fig. 3) simulate the histology. The cells vary markedly in size from 40 μ in Figure 4 to about 20 μ in diameter in Figure 11. Many of the cells show an ill-defined cytoplasm, but the nuclei are distinct and usually contain centrally placed acidophilic nucleoli. Angulations of the nuclear membrane are quite prominent (Figs. 3, 6, 7, 8, 14, 15, 16).

REFERENCES

1. Anderson WAD, Scotti TM: Synopsis of Pathology, ed. 8. St. Louis, MO:C. V. Mosby, Co., 1972.

126

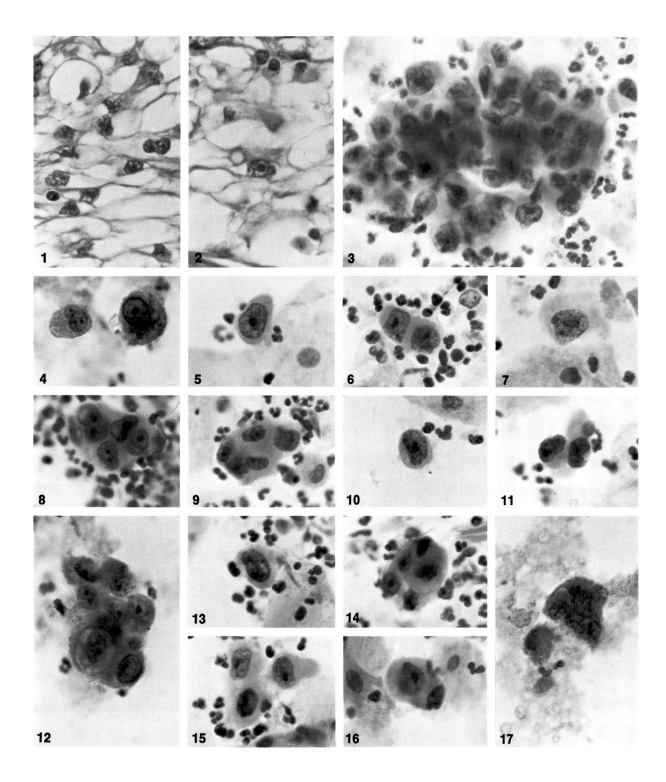

Plate 57

ADENOCARCINOMA, KIDNEY, METASTATIC TO LUNG

This 21-year-old female was ill for approximately six months, with debilitation and weight loss, and eventually developed a left supraclavicular lymphadenopathy. Concurrently, sputum studies were done, and X-ray of the chest revealed multiple nodules interpreted as metastatic tumor.

The section of a lymph node (Fig. 1) reveals complete replacement by tumor composed of glands lined by low cuboidal cells. These cells have clear cytoplasm and irregularly shaped nuclei with prominent acidophilic nucleoli.

The cells found in the sputum vary slightly in size and are seen as clusters or singly. Some of the cells appear to be very well preserved, similar to those in the sections (Figs. 2, 3, 9, 10), while others seem tightly packed, with dark nuclei that appear shrunken (Fig. 5, 6). All of the cells found in the smears are basophilically stained.

The histology and cytology suggested a clear cell pattern, and the primary site was suspected to be in the genital tract. Diethylstilbestrol exposure of the mother was not confirmed. Retrograde studies of the kidneys revealed a tumor of the left kidney.

128

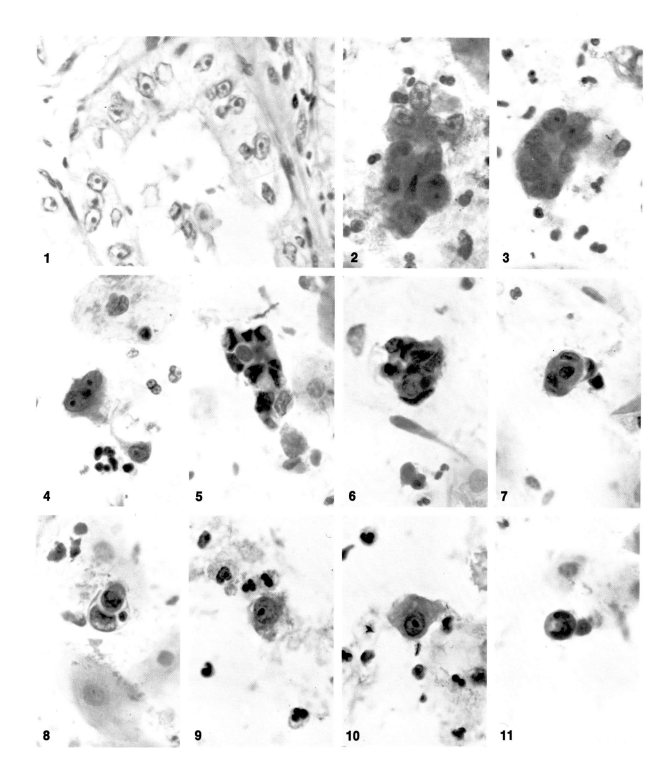

Plate 58

ADENOCARCINOMA OF LARGE BOWEL, METASTATIC TO LUNG

This patient was a 72-year-old male with adenocarcinoma of the large bowel with metastases to the liver. Adenocarcinoma of the large bowel frequently spreads locally or to the regional lymph nodes, metastasizes readily to the liver, and ultimately may metastasize to the lung. Some of the cells eventually are disseminated in the respiratory tree and found in sputum samples. When this happens, advanced disease with probably extensive carcinomatosis is indicated.

The cells found in the sputum measure 12–35 μ in diameter and are usually in clusters of several cells but may be single. These cells are not flat, and therefore it may be difficult to obtain a clear focus on all the cells in a cluster. These cells stain deeply basophilic. The nuclear/cytoplasmic ratio is increased, and pleomorphism is evident in all of the clusters, particularly those in Figures 4 and 5. The nuclear material is generally coarse and accumulates along the roughened wavy nuclear membrane (Figs. 2, 8, 10). Generally, these cells stand out in sputum smears because of clustering, hyperchromatism, and pleomorphism. It may be difficult to identify these as being of large bowel origin, but the features of staining and elongated nuclei suggest a gut origin for these cells. Of course, a clinical history of previous gut neoplasia is usually known, and the sputum study is to determine the extensiveness of the disease. It may indicate a serious state when the sputum is positive.

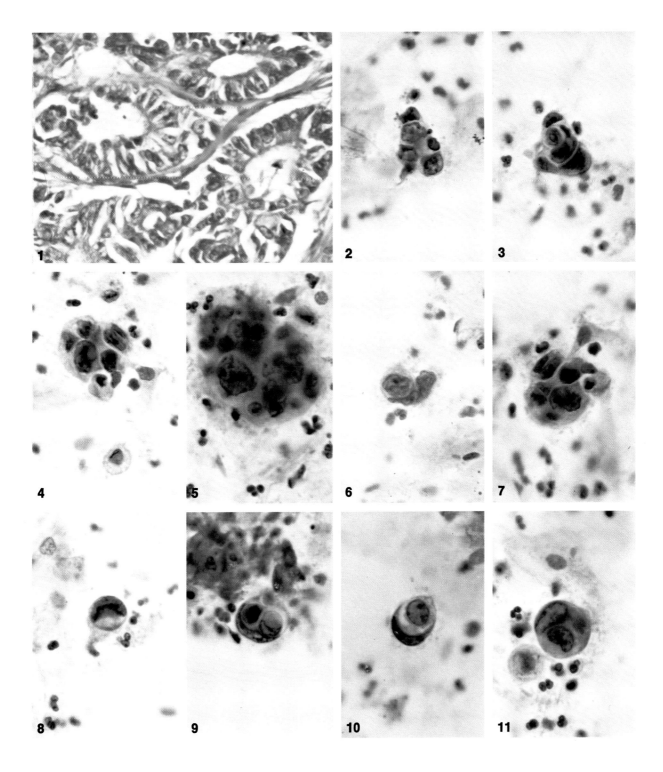

Plate 59

MELANOMA OF SKIN, METASTATIC TO LUNG

This tumor of the skin developed over the left scapula. It is a case of melanoma in a male 66 years of age. Melanoma is a tumor of all ages and a mimic of all tumors, and one must always remember these features. Metastatic lesions sometimes appear many years after the original diagnosis. In some cases, the patient will not even remember having a lesion removed. In the past, some skin lesions were discarded rather than sectioned for diagnosis. Since these tumors metastasize to the lymph nodes and lungs, enlarged nodes and lesions in the lung, which are difficult to diagnose or are considered suspicious histologically of melanoma, should be scrutinized for melanin. Even when the cells do not show melanin with H&E stain, a melanin stain sometimes will reveal this substance. A detailed clinical history should be obtained to determine if a skin lesion was removed previously.

Sections of tissue from the same areas of the tumor (Fig. 1) stained with H&E show only a slight yellowish tint in some of the cells, whereas in other sections (Fig. 2) an abundance of cytoplasmic melanin is present. Figure 3, stained for melanin, shows abundant melanin in spindle cells of the tumor. Figure 4 reveals abundant melanin in histiocytes in the sputum sample. Figures 5–10 depict melanotic tumor cells in the sputum. These are usually single (Figs. 7, 9, 10), but some clusters are also noted (Fig. 5). These cells are rather small (15–25 μ) and some show acidophilic nucleoli as seen in Figure 8. The nuclei contain coarse nuclear material, and the nuclear membrane is irregular and angled in most of these tumor cells.

132

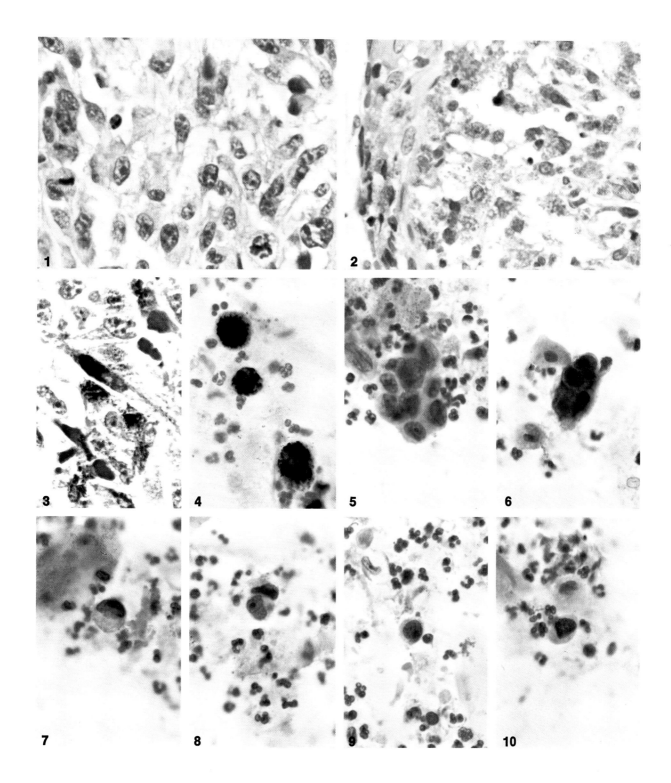

Plate 60

MELANOMA, METASTATIC TO LUNG

Primary melanoma of the bronchial tree is fortunately very rare but usually fatal because the diagnosis is difficult to make in the early stages of development. Metastases are early and usually fatal.

Metastatic melanoma to the lung usually has a poor prognosis. Often, one of the early signs of generalized metastasis is confirmed by melanoma cells in the sputum. These cells are often in clusters but may be single, measure from 20–60 μ in diameter, and usually are pigmented. If the cells do not contain menlanin, they may simulate mild metaplastic squamous cells, but study of the nuclei will reveal features of malignancy.

The melanin pigment in the cytoplasm of these cells is granular and has a yellowish cast, which aids in the differential identification from histiocytes. Sometimes histiocytes also engulf bile pigment and care should be taken to identify the pleomorphism of the neoplastic melanoma cells. Melanin stains[1] will also aid in the identification of these cells, sometimes revealing pigment even though the cells appear amelanotic with H&E stain. Usually these cells are not abundant but, when present, indicate the advanced degree of the tumor. Monitoring cases with sputum cytology and chemotherapy has been suggested by P. G. Moran (personal communication).

This case is of a 19-year-old female. Shown in this plate are a section of the metastatic tumor from the lung (Fig. 1) and the cells found in the sputum (Figs. 2–11).

REFERENCES

1. Bridges CH, Luna LG: Kerr's improved Warthin-Starry technic; study of the permissible variations. Lab Invest 6:356–367, 1957
2. Krementz ET, et al: Metastases of undetermined source. Ca 27:289–300, 1977

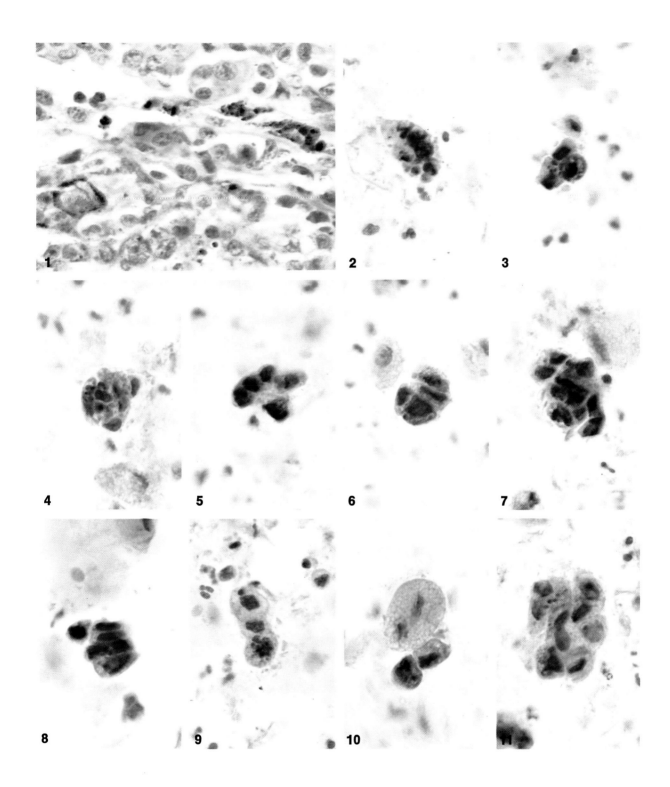

Plate 61

CARCINOMA, SQUAMOUS, LARYNX

Two cases are presented here. The first is of a 56-year-old male who smoked 20 cigarettes a day for 25 years and was diagnosed as having sputum cells considered positive for squamous cell carcinoma at age 53 (Fig. 2, 3). He had a normal chest X-ray and did not have a history of hemoptysis. No suggestive clinical symptoms were elicited except for a chronic cough. He had a fiberoptic bronchoscopy, which was entirely negative and was told no tumor was found. A year later, sputum cytology in connection with the Colorado uranium miner survey revealed many tumor cells (Figs 4–7). Another fiberoptic bronchoscopy was initiated, but the bronchoscopist noticed a small pale granular area on the margin of the left vocal cord, took a biopsy, and delayed the bronchoscopy pending results of the biopsy. The biopsy was positive (Fig. 1) for squamous cell carcinoma of the vocal cord. This was stripped and treated with cobalt, and the sputum has remained negative with no recurrence of the tumor. This tumor is a classical squamous cell carcinoma, grade II, and the cytology, as seen in Figures 2–7, shows large keratinizing, orangeophilic cells measuring 50 to over 100 μ in diameter. The nuclear/cytoplasmic ratio is increased in some of the cells (Figs. 2–4). This patient did not have hoarseness, and that is probably why the lesion was not detected at the first bronchoscopy. Possibly the lesion did not appear at the upper margin of the cord at that time.

The second case involves a 65-year-old male farmer who had smoked two packages of cigarettes a day for 40 years. His initial complaint was hoarseness, which at times caused complete aphonia. Laryngoscopy revealed no lesion of the vocal cords; however, laryngeal washings were done and these revealed nests of keratinized squamous cells consistent with tumor cells. The patient was admitted about three months later for laryngeal fissure. This was done, and extensive tumor involvement of both cords was found. A biopsy confirmed the diagnosis of squamous cell carcinoma, grade II (Figs. 8, 9), and a laryngectomy was done.

These two cases are different. One involved no clinical history of hoarseness, which always implies serious pathology of the larynx if present for more than a few weeks. This patient revealed positive sputum cytology with a visible lesion. The second case involved severe hoarseness with no visible lesion, but the sputum cytology (Figs. 10, 11) and wash were positive.

We have observed that in the presence of hoarseness, the cytology of a laryngeal wash or smears may not be identified as malignant but usually as marked atypia with normal nuclear/cytoplasmic ratio in most of the cells. Careful search, however, will eventually reveal nuclei which have coarse nuclear material, lobulations, crevices, etc. If hoarseness is present, then a direct view of the vocal cords should be obtained.

136

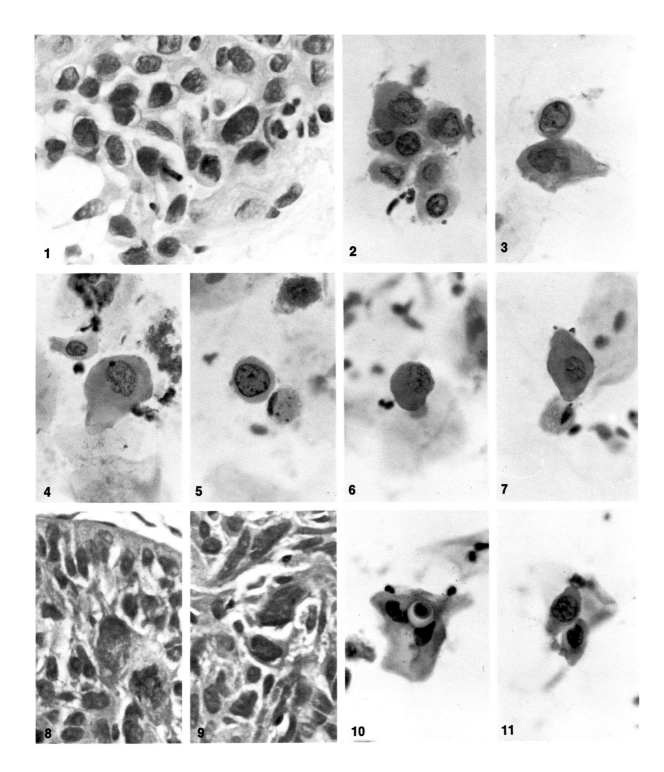

Plate 62

CARCINOMA, SQUAMOUS, KERATINIZING, LARYNX

A 67-year-old male was a cigarette smoker for many years and had sputum examinations on two occasions one year before surgery. Both examinations yielded results suggestive of malignancy (Figs. 2, 3). Careful examination with fiberoptic bronchoscopy revealed no abnormality. A year later, sputum studies again yielded a result positive for epidermoid carcinoma of the lung (Figs. 4–13). Laryngoscopy revealed a lesion of the left vocal cord, which was biopsied (Fig. 1), and a diagnosis of keratinizing squamous cell carcinoma was made. The cytology of this case shows unusually large masses of keratinizing cells (Figs. 2–6) and scattered single cells (Figs. 8–13). Large nuclei revealing coarse nuclear material with lobulations of nuclear substance and fissures of the nuclear membrane are also noted. The cytoplasm is abundant and very oran-geophilic. Most of the cells are very large, over 40–50 μ in diameter, but some smaller cells are also noted (Figs. 12, 13). This patient was successfully treated with cobalt and was free of symptoms after two years.

This is another example of a positive cytological examination of sputum identifying the presence of tumor, in the absence of hoarseness or clinical symptoms referable to the larynx. When the chest X-ray is negative, a careful examination of the larynx, particularly the vocal cords, should always be done if cytology of the sputum reveals malignant cells. A fiberoptic bronchoscopy should be performed only after examination of the larynx in suspected early lesions of the tracheobronchial tree.

138

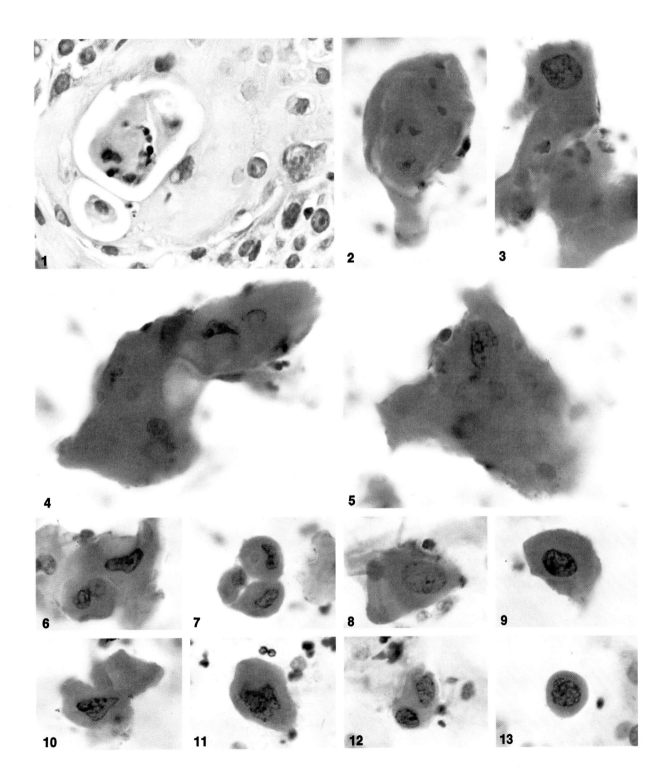

Plate 63

DEVELOPMENT OF EPIDERMOID CARCINOMA OF THE LUNG

Cancer of the lung, as mentioned previously, is an insidious disease which develops gradually over several years after prolonged exposure to carcinogens. This process takes about 10 to 20 years. Some writers believe and have presented rather convincing evidence that these tumors develop from metaplastic squamous cells, which replace normal tall columnar epithelia of the bronchial tree. These areas are small and most frequently seen at the spurs formed by dividing bronchi. Continued exposure to carcinogen or carcinogens causes an increasing atypia of these metaplastic cells, and eventually they develop into occult cancer and ultimately into frank invasive cancer.[1-4] Melamed[5] does not support this thesis and feels that the malignancy develops spontaneously from carcinogen-injured, but normal appearing, tall columnar epithelium. At this time, the exact mode of tumor development on exposure to carcinogens is not completely understood, is somewhat speculative, and deserves further study.

The first method of tumor development described above seems most reasonable for two reasons. First, squamous carcinomas of the lung are almost always bordered by areas of squamous cell metaplasia, which usually becomes more and more atypical as the tumor center is approached. Second, metaplastic cells found in sputum that have developed into moderate and marked atypical squamous cell metaplasia show increased DNA (polyploidy and heteroploidy), which is related to carcinogenesis.

Whether or not this theory will eventually be proven, one will always see, concomitant with tumor development, a gradual progression or ascending atypia of the metaplastic squamous cells, which almost predictably develop into neoplasia. These tumors develop similarly in cigarette smokers who are not miners and in cigarette smokers who mine uranium.

We have followed a large population of uranium miners for more than 20 years with annual sputum cytological studies. We have accumulated 38 cases that were followed for many years prior to development of malignancy of the lung, which was confirmed with histological diagnosis from node or tissue biopsy or from autopsy material. This plate shows 38 cases of confirmed cancer of the lung from this population. This chart, which is very informative about the epidemiology of this disease, shows that epidermoid lung cancer is a neoplasia of adulthood, with most cases occurring during the fourth, fifth, and sixth decades of life. The premalignant, atypical metaplastic stages varied considerably, as did the length of time of the carcinoma in situ. Some patients had double tumors. Some tumors were removed and the patients survived.

It should also be mentioned that the primary carcinogen in the uranium miners is cigarette smoking, which, when burdened with the additional carcinogen of radon daughters, increases the incidence of cancer of the lung. This disease is rare among the uranium miners who do not smoke cigarettes. This is also true of other non-cigarette smokers. A summary and average of the uranium miner population studied is presented in Plate 64.

REFERENCES

1. Auerbach O, et al: Changes in the bronchial epithelium in relation to smoking and cancer of the lung. N Engl J Med 256:97–104, 1957
2. Nasiell M: Metaplasia and atypical metaplasia in the bronchial epithelium: A histopathologic and cytopathologic study. Acta Cytol 10:421–427, 1966
3. Papanicolaou GN: A survey of actualities and potentialities of exfoliative cytology in cancer diagnosis. Ann Intern Med 31:661–674, 1949
4. Saccomanno G, et al: Development of carcinoma of the lung as reflected in exfoliated cells. CA 33:256–270, 1974
5. Melamed MR, et al: Radiologically occult in situ and incipient invasive epidermoid lung cancer. Am J Surg Pathol 1:5–16, 1977

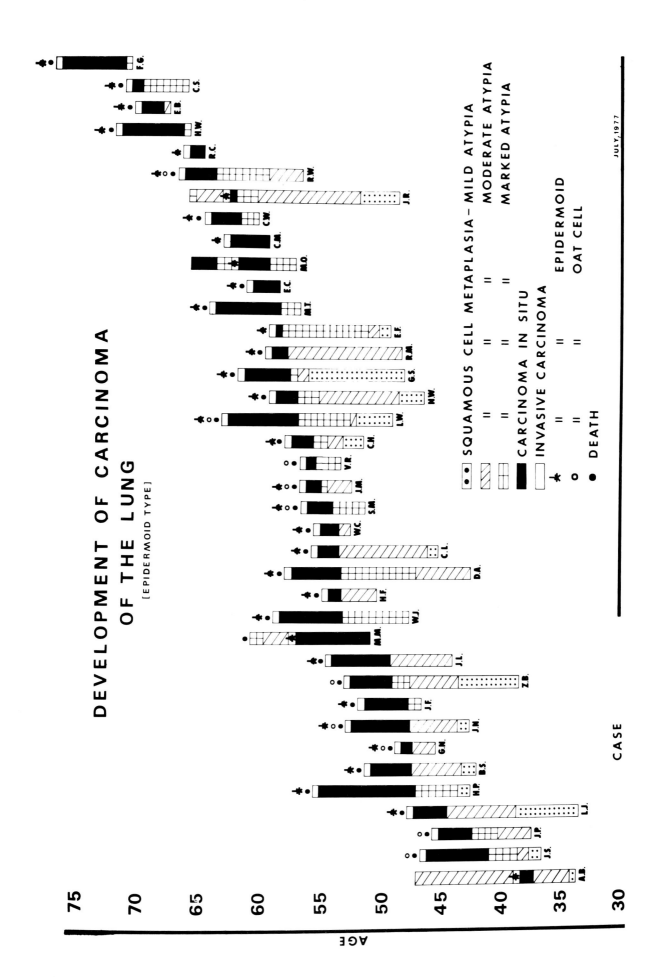

DEVELOPMENT OF CARCINOMA
OF THE LUNG
[EPIDERMOID TYPE]

SQUAMOUS CELL METAPLASIA – MILD ATYPIA
    "   "   =   MODERATE ATYPIA
    "   "   =   MARKED ATYPIA

CARCINOMA IN SITU   =   EPIDERMOID
INVASIVE CARCINOMA   =   OAT CELL

DEATH

CASE

AGE

JULY, 1977

(Modified from Saccomanno.[4])

Plate 64

DEVELOPMENT OF EPIDERMOID CARCINOMA OF THE LUNG— AVERAGE CASE

This graph presents an average of the data presented in Plate 63 on 33 of the 38 cases from the uranium miner study. It represents a summary of only 33 cases and, of course, these averages would be more significant and accurate if a larger sample of patients were available. Throughout the study, the various stages of development and the in-situ time period have not changed materially, so these results probably represent a rather reliable observation. The long period of the in-situ stage of epidermoid lung cancer (3.26 years) has been alluded to in the literature in single cases,[1-3] but has not been described as being of this time duration because the cases were not seen until they were more advanced. The time elapsed prior to diagnosis of neoplasia in these cases was, of course, impossible to ascertain. Too, there is a remote possibility that the life span of epidermoid lung cancer in the uranium miner may have a prolonged clinical course for some unknown reason, but this is an unlikely possibility since the clinical course, cytology, and histology of these tumors are not any different from this disease in the non-mining cigarette smokers. All possibilities must be considered.

Of course, the time period of the in-situ stage varies, as is noted in Plate 63, from less than a year to many years. This does indicate that sufficient time lag is available for localization of these lesions. With the methods presently under development, it seems very promising that these lesions will ultimately be localized very early, and a significant improvement in the five-year survival rate should be evident in the future treatment of this disease.

REFERENCES

1. Woolner LB, et al: In situ and early invasive bronchogenic carcinoma: Report of 28 cases with post operative survival data. J Thorac Cardiovasc Surg 60:275, 1970
2. Woolner LB Andersen A, Bernatz PE: "Occult" carcinoma of the bronchus: A study of 15 cases of in situ or early invasive bronchogenic carcinoma. Diseases of the Chest 37: 278–288, 1960
3. Papanicolaou GN, Koprawska I: Carcinoma in situ and right lower bronchus, case report. CA 4:141–146, 1951

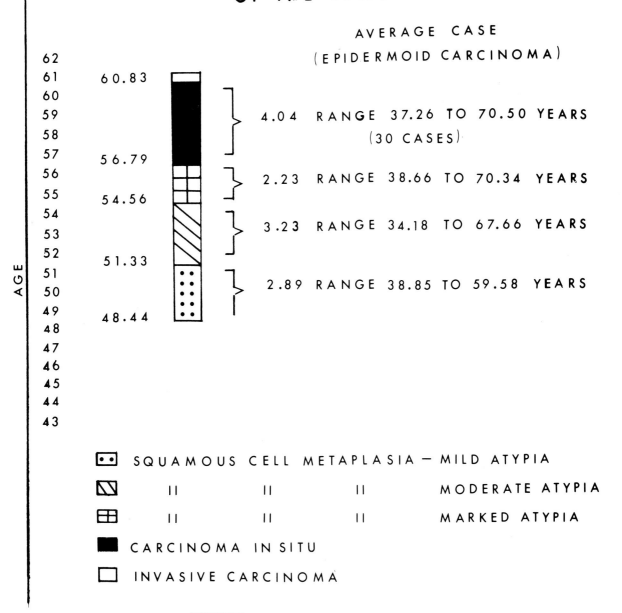

DEVELOPMENT OF CARCINOMA
OF THE LUNG

AVERAGE CASE
(EPIDERMOID CARCINOMA)

62
61   60.83
60
59   4.04   RANGE 37.26 TO 70.50 YEARS
58   (30 CASES)
57   56.79
56   2.23   RANGE 38.66 TO 70.34 YEARS
55   54.56
54
53   3.23   RANGE 34.18 TO 67.66 YEARS
52
51   51.33
50   2.89 RANGE 38.85 TO 59.58 YEARS
49   48.44
48
47
46
45
44
43

AGE

⊡ SQUAMOUS CELL METAPLASIA — MILD ATYPIA

◪   "   "   "   MODERATE ATYPIA

⊞   "   "   "   MARKED ATYPIA

■ CARCINOMA IN SITU

☐ INVASIVE CARCINOMA

Plate 65

PULMONARY CYTOLOGY

This chart is a summary of the results of sputum cytology performed at two hospitals with a combined bed capacity of 570. A number of cases involved outpatients, and the total number of samples examined was 4,000. Of these, 2,471 cases met the criteria for the analysis given here, which consisted of age and cigarette smoking history. All of the cases were referred for sputum cytology because of clinically suspected respiratory disease of one type or another. The sputum findings are recorded at the left; age, at the top of each column; and smoking (S) and nonsmoking (NS), at the base of each column. The totals (column at right) are a summary of each classification. At the bottom of the chart, a summary of each category of cell types is given in percentages of the total, with percent of smokers and nonsmokers beneath the total number of cases.

Assessment of the perpendicular columns reveals, first, that the majority of patients requiring sputum analysis were in their fourth through seventh decades of life. Second, it can be seen that the majority of the patients having sputum examinations were cigarette smokers, exceeding by far the smoking-nonsmoking ratio of 75.68% vs. 24.32%. Horizontal examination of the abnormal cases reveals that the majority of patients were found to show a mild atypical squamous cell metaplasia. This degree of cellular change is usually due to respiratory infections. Moderate atypia is the next most frequent, particularly in the fifth through seventh decades. This may be a product primarily of cigarette smoking. The marked atypical squamous cell metaplasia is not much higher than the number of primary lung neoplasias, which are most numerous in the sixth and seventh decades and most of these were in the cigarette smoking columns. The majority of patients with positive metastatic sputa were in their sixth and seventh decades.

144

PULMONARY CYTOLOGY

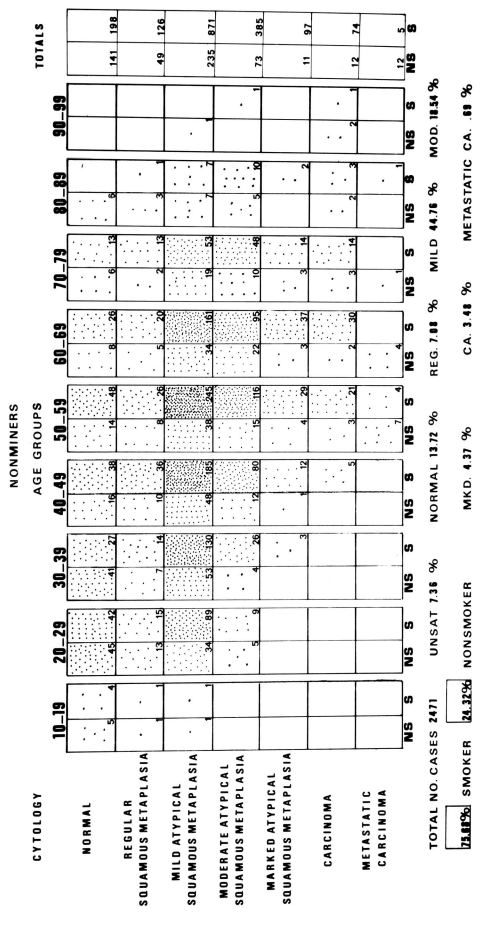

NONMINERS

AGE GROUPS

TOTAL NO. CASES 2471

SMOKER 75.88% NONSMOKER 24.32%

UNSAT 7.36 %   NORMAL 13.72 %   REG. 7.08 %   MILD 44.76 %   MOD. 18.54 %

MKD. 4.37 %   CA. 3.48 %   METASTATIC CA. .69 %

INDEX

146